1991

AIDS
Sharing the Pain

AIDS
Sharing the Pain

A GUIDE FOR CAREGIVERS

Bill Kirkpatrick

Foreword by
William A. Doubleday

The Pilgrim Press
NEW YORK

This book is dedicated to
all whose courage of love
enables me to share their pain
as I attempt to be alongside them

All royalties from the sale of this volume are being given to CRUSAID,
an organization for those living with HIV and AIDS.

Library of Congress Cataloging-in-Publication Data

Kirkpatrick, Bill.
AIDS, sharing the pain : a guide for caregivers / Bill Kirkpatrick
: foreword by William A. Doubleday.
p.   cm.
Includes bibliographical references.
ISBN 0-8298-0827-2
1. AIDS (Disease)—Psychological aspects.   I. Title.
RC607.A26K57   1990
362.1′969792—dc20   89-22997

The Pilgrim Press, 475 Riverside Dr., New York, N.Y. 10115

Contents

Foreword to the American Edition

Early in the AIDS epidemic, most Americans had a simplistic view of the illness and its sufferers. People with AIDS were branded as "victims." Treatment options were few and largely ineffectual. Long-term survival was unknown. AFRAIDS (Acute Fear Regarding AIDS) was spreading even faster than the AIDS illness itself.

Change has come slowly. Today we hear many people talking about "living with AIDS"; we read about a growing number of long-term AIDS survivors; we learn how HIV infection may span many years of a lifetime. Just as cancer is no longer accepted as an inevitable or immediate death sentence in our society, so too AIDS has become a challenge to battle, an occasion for healing, an invitation to explore or engage every spiritual resource the church, our culture, or any individual can muster into service.

Clearly, it is no longer sufficient to think of AIDS as a predictable set of symptoms, an inevitable course of illness, or an invariably rapid or certain cause of death. Today, more than ever before, the AIDS epidemic raises a broad spectrum of life situations with a wide range of pastoral and spiritual implications. Simplistic stereotyping has sometimes caused us to miss the nuances and complexity of the impact of the AIDS illness on diverse and inevitably unique individuals. The predominant demographics of the epidemic in particular parts of the country, the makeup of our caseloads, and our ability to identify with certain of the so-called risk groups for AIDS have all contributed to our vision or blindness about who has AIDS, what their illness is like, and what their needs may be in terms of our caring response.

Today AIDS is about "the worried well" and "the HIV antibody positive." AIDS is about people living with AIDS and about the need for hospice-type services for those who are finally dying from it. AIDS is about hemophiliacs and transfusion recipients, women and children, prisoners and prostitutes. AIDS can be about disfigurement or dementia, about hunger or homelessness, about depression or despair. AIDS is about drug treatment programs and sex education for young and old, straight and gay. AIDS is still too often about rejection and neglect by families, friends, employers, or health and social service workers. AIDS has too often been about rejection and neglect by the churches and clergy of this land.

Indeed, problems often arise when religious groups, having taken the position that they cannot or must not condone certain behaviors that their particular tradition considers to be "immoral," nonetheless feel a strong scriptural mandate to carry out "works of mercy" for the sick, the suffering, and the dying. Experience suggests that every religious tradition has pastors, counselors, and chaplains who are able to minister with compassion and sensitivity, as well as those who will almost certainly deliver a message of guilt, judgment, or outright condemnation. It is clear, of course, that people who are sick, dying, or bereaved should be shielded as much as possible from proselytizing, judgmentalism, or intrusion on their desired privacy.

One of the pioneers in the compassionate pastoral response to the AIDS crisis in the United Kingdom was Bill Kirkpatrick, an Anglican priest who has long been involved in ministry to those on the margins of church and society in London. This book is written out of Kirkpatrick's pastoral experience on the English scene. It is wise, sensible, and compassionate toward all sorts and conditions of men and women. It tends to focus mainly upon the gay male sufferers of AIDS. Indeed, they will continue to be the people with AIDS most likely to be encountered by most American clergy. The book does not pretend to address in detail the particularly difficult issues of AIDS among the urban poor in America, a circumstance severely compounded by issues of addiction, racism, and economic injustice. We may hope that a book addressing those particular challenges will emerge in the near future.

What this book does very well is to communicate a common-sense approach to pastoral care that is utterly compassionate and thoroughly rooted in the gospel of love. If you are starting out in AIDS ministry it will guide and inspire you. If you are a veteran on the edge of burn-out, you will be heartened to hear things you have been trying to say yourself.

The Rev. William A. Doubleday
General Theological Seminary
New York
Independence Day 1989

Preface

This book is for all the men and women who, whether they are ordained or not, minister to those living and suffering through the evolving stages of HIV infection, loosely called AIDS. In writing for this particular caring group, I am fully aware of the many who are not ordained—men and women who are, if you like, the backbone of all pastoral care, Christian and non-Christian alike. I include of course all those living with this viral infection and its consequences who minister to each other and to the caring team.

My caring has been mainly with members of the gay community simply because in this country they are at present the largest group of persons affected. *This does not mean that I am unaware of the fact that worldwide the largest group affected is heterosexual.* I am also of course aware of those other groups: drug users infected through the sharing of needles; prostitutes, male and female, whose activities make them especially vulnerable; those infected through being sexually abused; those infected through blood transfusion; those in prison; babies and young children who have been infected through their mothers' infection, whatever its source; the many thousands in the third world where the infection rate is devastatingly high.

I write through the truth of my experience of sharing the pain and the courage of all who have allowed me 'to be' alongside them, whether in the hospital or their community; not only with those persons who are infected but also with others who, like myself, are attempting to care and who are so often in need of supportive care themselves. It is through this sharing, unconditionally from a non-judgemental stance, that the large 'C' of compassion is being put back into the work of caring. As a result medical and other models within the caring professions are rethinking their position towards alternative forms of medical, psychological and social care.

No one writes a book on his or her own. The author dares to be the public spokesperson for those who are its source of inspiration. In truth, it has been written for me by all those unique individuals who are infected; and also by their partners, families and friends and all those who care for them through their own need to care and be cared for.

I cannot begin to name the many individuals who are in the heart of this book by an author whose life will never be the same again. Yet there are those who have especially had the courage to set time aside, each in their own individual ways, to share in its writing, although I alone am responsible for its imperfections, as well as everything else.

My thanks to: Lesley Riddle, of Darton, Longman and Todd, who had the courage of faith to invite me to put pen to paper; Tony and Robina Masters who helped sort out my scribbles, strange words and the punctuation; Richie McMullen, not only for his generosity in allowing his very personal 'inside the pain' story to be shared, but for his other contributions towards improving this book; Elizabeth Goodrum who found herself constantly retyping my scratch marks; Bishop Mark Santer for his Foreword and his constant support of those involved in the AIDS ministry; Rev. William Doubleday for his Foreword to the American edition; Dr. Charles Farthing, Research Registrar in AIDS at St Stephen's Hospital, Chelsea, who sorted out the medical notes: Dr and Mrs Paul Clarke, Verena Tschudin and Heather Snidle whose comments on the manuscript have enriched the book; Peter Randall whose discussions with me in the past two years confirmed me in my growing awareness of my being outside the pain of being antibody positive; Bernard Hughes, Barry Newton, and David Brown, hospital chaplains whose experiences parallel mine; Tony Whitehead who has encouraged and supported me in this growing area of need; the many men and women who are living, suffering and dying because of this new viral infection; those whom I knew and are now living beyond the dimension of this life, but are linked with us forever through the embrace of love's unendingness. It is they rather than myself who have written this book for all who attempt to care and be cared for as together we live out 'the least you offer to one of these my brothers and sisters, you are offering to me' from within the faith of love's endeavouring.

Bill Kirkpatrick
London

Introduction:
Healing Wounds Mutually Shared

This book sets out some guidelines for the pastoral care of all who suffer from Human Immunodeficiency Virus (HIV). In doing so, it ranges in subject from a brief history and definition of the disease itself to an analysis of pastoral care from within the services of faith, hope and love, and to the material practicalities of organisations and resources which are available to help antibody positive persons and carers alike. Everyone must be encouraged to realise that, for the AB+ persons, it is the *quality* of their life that has now become important rather than its length. This quality can be enhanced or affected through the mystery of compassionate caring shared mutually by all, including those who are antibody positive.

This book does not attempt to moralise or to examine in detail the medical cause and effect of HIV infection. Rather, it sets out to show how to bring a positive approach, with confidence and fresh hope, not only to those infected with this new virus but also to their partners, families and friends. My approach has nothing to do with the wrath of God but *everything* to do with the love of God for each and every person.

As the awareness of HIV infection grows so do the ignorance and the fears and prejudices of society, despite the educational campaigns of voluntary groups and the government. As a result, pastoral care has become increasingly important for persons living with HIV (PLW-HIV), their partners, families, friends and society alike.

It is essential that ministers and other carers should be unafraid and knowledgeable about this viral infection and its pattern of action. For this reason, it is vital for such carers to keep up to date with the latest *authentic* information about the disease and the various treatments available.

In addition, it is essential for us all to be aware of the different choices of action available to combat the infection mentally, physically, socially and spiritually according to the specific needs of each person. We should feel free enough to share information on how to cope with the practical and sometimes burdensome issues of living: the daily expenses and the income needs; home help needs; accommodation needs; work needs; social and spiritual needs. We must know how to obtain legal help as well as assistance from the statutory services and about the help available from the various supportive voluntary groups. Counsellors and helpers need to be well informed about the large amount of legal and practical resources available.

In our attempts to offer realistic pastoral care, we need to be aware of the hidden, in-depth feelings of the person who is caught up in the mysteries (the different stages) of this infection. Generally, the first reaction to the knowledge of HIV infection is one of shock, of disbelief and a growing anxiety about the progress of the infection and of the real possibility of his or her eventual death. The anxiety is made more acute by the projection of fears about losing his or her physical or mental faculties during the progression of the infection.

In my experience, those who are infected and those who share their suffering need someone to be with them on *their* terms as they try to find a real meaning in a life which is now being viewed as, and felt by themselves to be, meaningless.

This viral disease has repercussions for everyone. It tests the sincerity of our acceptance of the person; of our commitment to our relationship with him or her; of our commitment of compassion for the sufferer and the quality of our faith.

As carers, it is essential for us to be aware of our own feelings, values and moral outlook while realising that the PLW-HIV's views may be very different from ours. This is so because, while he or she is *in* the disease, we are always *outside* it. Only when this distinction has been mutually accepted is there a basis for the beginning of a stronger bonding between carer and PLW-HIV. At all times carers must be non-judgemental listeners who hear, who feel and yet who are positive and honest with this person about each stage of the illness. The same considerations must apply also to our pastoral care of the partner and/or lover and their respective families and friends.

It is essential for us to recognise that, at present, PLW-HIV (who may or may not have an early death) and those who are close to them are being made to face up to their own mortality. For the sufferer, there is also the spectre of facing two deaths. First, the possible 'death' of 'coming out' and of facing his or her homosexuality (and, for some, their bisexuality) with all the shame, guilt and rejection that society and the Church has invested this with. Secondly, he or she has to come to terms with the actuality of impending physical and mental disability leading to death and the manner of his or her death and when this may take place.

In addition, the infected person has three other major fears: of loneliness, of pain and a feeling of uselessness. Those who are antibody positive need to know that they will not be abandoned or rejected. Similarly, those who are dying from this disease need the constant assurance that they will be as free as possible from pain; that they will die with the dignity of being loved, and of being supported and surrounded by the most important people in their lives. They will want to share and to express their love and to be assured that it will be recognised and accepted for what it is and on its own terms as they search for the answers to the deepest questions that they may ever have faced:

'How am I going to die?'
'What will happen to me when I die?'
'Am I acceptable to God?'

What all persons need is a genuine authentication of themselves as being of value – even in their dying. The PLW-HIV, like his socially stigmatised predecessor the leper, may ask, 'Is the Church a centre of listening for *all* people?' As pastoral carers, we have to prove that it is a centre of listening for *all*. The Christian response to this crisis of infection in all its stages should not be judgemental or fearful but compassionate, and we should remember that every sufferer is Jesus in painful disguise, indeed is all of us in painful disguise.

In our caring, we must be ready to accompany the person on his or her unique pilgrimage through the different stages of the disease which may lead to his or her death. The various psychological stages of dying which most of us will go through are denial, anger, bargaining, depression, acceptance and then waiting.

It is important for ministers and others offering pastoral care to be aware of and accept these various psychological states, which we may see manifested in different people or even the same person within the space of a few hours.

In order to help such people, we need to be psychologically comfortable with our own suffering; our own fears of contagion and infection; our own sexuality (a great problem for many Christians) and our own mortality. To deny any emotional connection with the person is to increase the physical, psychological, social and spiritual violence of the disease. We must always be prepared to ask ourselves, 'Have I the courage of faith to recognise myself and to *be with* this person according to his or her needs and in line with his or her perceptions, which are themselves in a constant state of flux?'

It is crucial for us to realise that while we may share in the person's pain, we cannot actively feel or take on the uniqueness of the pain. When we recognise this limitation, then the barriers of professionalism vanish and we are no longer afraid of our mutual humanness. By looking at our own frailties, our own vulnerabilities and coming to realise and understand their creative potential, we are released into a mode of being with the other person, a mode of being that allows us to embrace him or her in such a way that *their* total involvement in the disease can become also a release for *them* in ways that are not only co-creative but also co-healing for all concerned.

Whenever I use the prefix 'co' meaning 'together' before the words 'creative' and 'healing', I am stressing the fact that we do nothing of our own, however much it may outwardly appear that we do. 'Where two or more are gathered in my name . . . I Jesus am present and my name is Love.'* In all pastoral caring there is the person seeking and there is the person offering and there is that 'mysterious other' that brings them together.

This new viral infection reminds us that all new diseases are a mystery, just as death is, and we are angry and helpless, often enraged at our impotence. It is vital that we acknowledge this helplessness, that we do not deny it but rather 'own it' fully. This acceptance of our own emotional range has particular significance for carers participating in the experience of a ministry which is being shared with all suffering persons.

We should also be aware that we are being ministered to as we grow with these sufferers, and through them, in our Christian understanding of death and its deathlessness. In the light of Christ's death and resurrection, his ultimate healing, this death and deathlessness increases its meaning for us. In each person, as in all of us, there are the seeds of our innate healing potential.

The minister comes (as do other carers) to the pastoral caring situation as a person rich in the kind of faith, hope and love that nourishes one's ability to grow into the mystery of shared compassion and allows for the mutual embrace of sufferer and carer alike. The priest is ordained to be central in sharing in the pain of others. He or she is ordained to be with this person, humanising the embrace of God's love towards all his people in all those personal and other situations where suffering and healing meet. Increasingly, I am being shown how to be in this area of suffering not only by those who are antibody positive but also by their lovers, families and friends who are suffering with them.

It is quite impossible to put into words the immense difficulties which all carers will face. The following is the third reading from the Body Positive Memorial Service 1987 and it expresses many of them. It was written by Dietmar Bolle, a nurse caring for others and, like them, suffering himself from HIV infection.

* Mt. 18:20.

I want to cry
for people and friends
and lovers and all those
whom I have loved and nursed
and nursed and loved
and who have gone to sleep
and left me to go on
to give strength to all the others
who are left alone
and sometimes it feels like
I carry the burden of the whole world
on my shoulders.

I feel as if I can't go on any more
that everything is too much
but, then, from time to time,
somebody comes up to me
and reassures me again:
'You know,' he says, 'only your
presence alone gives enough strength
to go on or to find a way to come to peace
with oneself.'

And I sit at one's bed and think:
Who is the one who gives?
And then I want to cry
for those who feel so alone
for those who committed suicide
for those who have been closest of all to me
without knowing it.

And for all the others
I have never met:
'Sleep well.
Maybe I'll see you again
sometime
but please, don't wait for me.
I want to stay here
for quite a while.'

2

The Dis-ease of Disease:
A Brief History

During the early part of 1981, the first signs that a *new* viral infection had occurred was the admission of five young men to various hospitals in Los Angeles. They were suffering from a rare type of pneumonia caused by a commonly occurring protozoa known as *pneumocystis carinii*, previously only seen in patients whose immune systems had become deficient due to other causes.

At about the same time in New York City, physicians were reporting on the occurrence of a severe form of *Kaposi's sarcoma* in a group of young men. This sarcoma takes the form of a tumour of blood vessel tissue in the skin and/or the internal organs. It was previously known to occur among elderly Italian and Jewish men. What these otherwise healthy young men had in common was that they all had evidence of *immunodeficiency* not related to any known cause, and several also had other serious infections. All were homosexual, ranging in age from twenty to fifty years, the mean age being between thirty and thirty-five. It was towards the end of 1981 that the first man diagnosed as suffering from AIDS was seen in a London hospital.

Although AIDS was first recognised in the USA and the UK among male homosexuals, it became clear in the early months that AIDS was not confined specifically to this group of people even though most of the men diagnosed as being infected with the HIV virus were either homosexual or bisexual. Also at risk were the intravenous substance abusers (i.e. drug addicts), persons with haemophilia, the heterosexual partners of persons with AIDS or at risk of AIDS, recipients of transfused blood or blood components, and

7

children from families in which one or both parents are HIV infected.

The risk of developing AIDS varies in different parts of the world. At present in the West, the major 'at risk' groups are homosexual and bisexual men, intravenous substance abusers and prostitutes. In Central Africa, where the infection is an epidemic involving millions of lives, homosexuals do not make up a significant number of people with AIDS. In Africa, the major 'at risk' group is *all* sexually active individuals, especially in towns, cities and those villages that border major trucking routes across the African continent.

In fact, all who are leading a sexually active life are at serious risk. This does not mean to say you have to be promiscuous to be infected; a *single encounter* with an infected person could lead to being infected with the virus.

Definition of the disease

The definition of AIDS was first outlined by the Communicable Disease Centre (CDC) in Atlanta, Georgia, USA, in 1982. Its definition was precise and highly specific: a reliably diagnosed disease suggestive of a defect in cell mediated immunity in a person with *no known* cause for the immunity. The virus was not known in 1982.

Since the introduction of blood tests in 1985 which can detect whether or not the person has been *exposed* to the AIDS virus (the Human Immunodeficiency Virus or HIV), the definition has changed to 'the occurrence of a disease suggestive of a cell mediated immunity in a person with no known cause for that condition other than HIV'. It is the homosexual community that has, in the main, taken the brunt of the new viral infection in the West, simply because, by an accident of history, here in the West the HIV was introduced first into this community. (For the current definition of AIDS, see the end of this chapter.)

The bare facts

This book offers pastoral guidelines to ministers and other carers rather than a detailed account of the disease and its

8

medical treatment. Nevertheless it is essential that we are aware of what I call the 'bare facts of HIV infection', as these are basic to all who are concerned with being alongside the sufferer and those who suffer with him or her.

I write about 'HIV infection' rather than of AIDS itself because I believe that initially this is the condition we are attempting to understand. When we talk about AIDS, we are talking about the terminal result of having been infected with HIV. I therefore believe it to be more correct to talk of HIV infection rather than of AIDS, not least because it does leave some hope for those infected of not progressing mentally, even if they do so physically, into the terminal potential of this viral infection.

HIV infection is the result of being infected with a new virus – Human Immunodeficiency Virus – which can result in the person developing what is commonly known as AIDS, often called 'Frank AIDS' or 'Full-blown AIDS'. This virus weakens the immune system, causing the body to be more susceptible to opportunistic infections. So far it is not known how many of those who are 'antibody positive' will proceed to develop AIDS itself.

Seropositive-testing for infection is done by looking for HIV antibodies which may be present in the blood. These are protein molecules that the body makes in an effort, usually unsuccessful, to defeat the virus. If the antibodies are found, the person is said to be 'HIV antibody positive' or 'body positive'. This does not mean that the person has AIDS, but it does mean that he or she carries the virus and is at risk of developing AIDS itself.

The development from the infection to AIDS

The development from the initial HIV infection to AIDS itself usually occurs through different stages and at differing rates of speed. The following is a brief synopsis of these stages:

1 *Initial HIV infection*
Within a few weeks (and occasionally within a few hours) of the virus entering the body, some people experience something which may resemble influenza or glandular fever. This

9

is usually followed by a long period when the disease is entirely latent. During this period, the infected person may feel completely well and yet be infectious to others. It is because of this quiet period that the infection may remain undetected for many years and why this particular viral infection poses such a threat towards *all* who are sexually active, as infected people may unwittingly be passing on the virus.

2 *Persistent generalised Lymphadenopathy (PGL)*
During this phase, there is a general swelling of the lymph nodes or glands caused by the activity of this virus. These swellings may last for long periods of time. The patient may or may not be aware of the swollen glands.

3 *AIDS related complex (ARC)*
The HIV virus has, by now, severely damaged the natural immune system. The symptoms are often milder and less specific than for those suffering from AIDS itself. The person affected may be suffering from night sweats, fevers, severe malaise, fatigue, lethargy, excessive loss of weight, persistent diarrhoea, skin rashes, etc. It is important to realise that, at this stage, he or she can sometimes be more ill than someone with 'Full-blown AIDS' and may well be in need of a great deal of care and support.

4 *AIDS dementia complex (ADC)*
This is caused by an invasion by the virus of the central nervous system, especially of the brain, due to HIV having passed through the blood-brain barrier, which usually filters out substances in the blood which may damage the brain. Should this occur, then the person may suffer confusion, memory loss and difficulty in walking, and may require complete bodily and social care for the rest of his or her life.

5 *Full-blown AIDS*
Full-blown AIDS, also known as 'Frank AIDS', is the ultimate indication that the immune system is collapsing as, by this time, the body has been attacked by at least one life-threatening opportunistic infection or tumour. The AIDS

virus causes damage in an indirect way by destroying the ability of the body to resist or control infection.

The letters A–I–D–S spell out for us the basic facts of this infection:

(a) It is an *Acquired* infection, meaning that one is not usually born with the problem.

(b) It attacks the body's *Immune* system, i.e. the body's natural defence system – causing

(c) *Deficiency* of operation, leaving the body vulnerable to a whole host of other infections known as 'opportunistic infections'.

(d) It is recognised by the occurrence of one or several of a group of diseases known collectively as a *Syndrome*.

A–cquired, i.e. generallly not born with
I–mmune, i.e. to do with the body's defence system
D–eficiency, i.e. deficiency of that system
S–yndrome, i.e. a group of diseases

Who may be infected?

1 All those who are involved in sexual practices with an infected person, the most dangerous being penetrative and/or vaginal intercourse.

2 All intravenous drug abusers who share their used equipment with other users who are infected with HIV.

3 Babies of infected mothers are susceptible to being infected *in utero* and possibly also through mother's milk while breast-feeding.

4 All those persons who have received infected blood transfusions, or blood products, such as factor 8, which are used for haemophilia. This is extremely rare now that all blood products are being heat-treated and all blood tested for antibodies.

It is essential for all concerned to realise, and to accept the fact, that HIV is extremely virulent in the body but is one of the weakest outside the body. Away from the warm bodily fluids, it is very easily destroyed by ordinary household bleach or by soap. The virus has a fatty membrane as an outer coat which is easily destroyed by detergents.

11

You cannot be infected with HIV from:
1 Casual contacts: shaking hands, touching, hugging, dry kissing or sharing a bed.
2 Sneezing and coughing (it is not an airborne disease) or minor abrasions or giving blood.
3 The use of glasses, cups, knives, forks, spoons, cooking utensils, toilet seats, showers, swimming pools.
4 Sharing books, newspapers, pencils, biros or any other inanimate object.

You can avoid being infected with the HIV virus by:
1 Remembering that one does not have to be promiscuous to become infected.
2 Avoiding risky vaginal or anal intercourse. Penetrative intercourse can be made relatively safe by the use of condoms, but there is still some risk, however, as condoms may break. The use of water-soluble lubricants (preferably containing spermicides as these are toxic to the virus) will lessen the chances of the condom breaking. Do *not* use oil-based lubricants, as these weaken the rubber of the condom.
3 Not sharing unclean needles or syringes if you are an intravenous drug abuser.
4 Not losing control via excessive drinking or other forms of drug taking.

If anyone is in doubt as to whether he or she may or may not be antibody positive, then the only course of action is to seek advice and counselling about having an antibody test. *It is not the function of the minister or any other caring person to decide for the person involved – it must be his or her own decision.* The carer's responsibility is to be alongside him or her whatever the decision and the subsequent outcome of the test.

When talking about HIV infection

When talking about HIV infection, we should do so in such a way as to alleviate many of the fears not only of those who are infected and those who suffer with them, but also of the great majority of people known as 'the worried well'. The following statements may enable us to talk more positively and thereby lessen the fears so often founded upon untruths.

1 We should be talking about HIV infection rather than about AIDS, because many who are currently infected have not moved into the most vulnerable area of this infection, i.e. 'Full-blown AIDS'.

2 We should be talking about the person 'living with' rather than 'dying of' this viral infection.

3 We should be talking about 'the person with HIV infection' rather than the 'patient'. The person becomes a 'victim' through the leperisation tactics of fear, rather than through any disease.

4 We should be talking about a 'life-threatening' illness rather than a 'terminal' one. The perception of this disease as an inevitable death sentence leaves the person without any hope and says much more about our attitudes to disease and death than about the disease itself. It is important to realise that no one, strictly speaking, dies of AIDS itself. The different causes of death are directly related to the person's depressed immune system which is unable to combat the various opportunistic infections which attack it.

5 We should be talking about 'risk activities' rather than about 'risk groups' because *all* sexually active persons are 'at risk' where 'safer sex' practices are not the norm.

6 We should be talking about this disease as being the 'result of an infection by a new virus'. Like all diseases, it can be fought and *is* being fought on behalf of the millions of men, women and children who are suffering as a result of this viral infection throughout the world today.

The current definition of AIDS itself is: 'The occurrence of a disease suggestive of a defect in cell mediated immunity occurring in a person with no known cause for diminished immunity other than the presence of HIV.'

The diseases accepted as being 'suggestive' of such a defect are strictly listed and include:

Pneumocystis carinii pneumonia (proven or presumptive)
Toxoplasma cerebral abscesses
Cryptosporidial diarrhoea (for longer than a month)
Cytomegalovirus: retinitis, enterocolitis, pneumonitis or encephalitis

Progressive long lasting herpes
Candidal (thrush) oesophagitis
Cryptococcal (fungal) meningitis
Disseminated atypical mycobacterial (TB) disease
Severe chronic loss of weight
Encephalopathy/Myelopathy (brain or spinal cord disease),
secondary to HIV itself
Kaposi's sarcoma
Non Hodgkin's lymphoma (a tumour of the lymph glands)

AIDS has been called 'the opportunistic disease of society'.
It can also be seen to be the 'opportunistic disease of the
Body of Christ'. It is an opportunity to be compassionate
towards all who suffer in our world of imperfect societies.
When it does this, it is saying that all who have died or who
are suffering because of this disease have made, and are
making, an invaluable contribution towards the healing of all
humanity.

I should like to re-emphasise the following important
points:

1 It has now been established that AIDS is by no means
confined to the homosexual community.

2 All sexually active persons are at risk when safer sex
practices are not the norm.

3 We cannot moralise or be judgemental towards any infection however mild or severe.

4 This is not a heaven-sent plague imposed by God, but a
menacing and virulent virus that has emerged quite naturally
and for which we must believe an eventual cure will be found.

5 HIV infection has a kind of leprosy aura about it and
presents ministers with practical and moral problems very
similar to those presented by the lepers to Jesus. Yet he did
not turn his back on them; neither should we turn our backs
on those who are suffering from this new viral infection.

3

AFRAIDS

Love casts out all fear

During a visit to the USA and Canada in 1986, I found that
many were talking about an even greater disease than AIDS,
which is affecting the person infected, those who are suffering
with him or her, and those who are the 'worried well'. It is the
disease known as 'AFRAIDS' – that is 'Acute Fear Regarding
AIDS'. This is succinctly recorded by William A Doubleday
in his essay 'Spiritual and Religious Issues of AIDS':

> The religious community is well aware of the existence of
> two epidemics, AIDS and what the magazine *New Republic*
> has named AFRAIDS (Acute Fear Regarding AIDS).
> While medical science tells us that AIDS itself is not casu-
> ally transmitted, AFRAIDS, unfortunately, is too casually
> transmitted by gossip, jokes, graffiti, sensationalist news
> and entertainment media and some politically, socially and
> theologically conservative TV and radio evangelists. While
> AIDS sufferers usually benefit from pastoral care, the
> anxieties of AFRAIDS sufferers are often aggravated by
> misguided religious professionals who could be countering
> AFRAIDS with pastoral care, education, and the setting
> of a compassionate example. The task of the religious
> community in responding to the AFRAIDS crisis is
> compounded by the fact that while AIDS is unfortunately
> almost invariably fatal within a few years, AFRAIDS
> thrives on closed minds and hearts and may last for an
> unshortened lifetime. Many more millions are afflicted with

AFRAIDS than carry antibodies to the AIDS virus in their blood.*

What is required of priests and other caring persons is an *open* mind to the real facts of this viral infection. Such openness of mind will allow for responsible safer sex education and practices which are not only procreative but also co-creative in this most sacred of shared human activities. One of our main functions as ministers and carers is to educate and, through this educative function, enable the fearful to understand the source of their fears. Such education may be of a factual kind and fear may be dispelled through sharing a terminology that is applicable to each group. The openness of a fearless mind will reveal that AFRAIDS is born of unfounded fears nourished through fear breeding fear.

Somehow the nature of this particular disease arouses fears, very basic fears, in most people's lives. Such fears include: fear of the unknown, fear of infection and contagion, fear of sexual activity and fear of our own mortality.

The Surgeon General of the United States of America has constantly said, loudly and clearly, that our main protection against infection and a further spread of the disease (until a vaccine can be developed and made available to *all*) is informed education. All must be kept informed, especially those who are sexually active.

This is why the minister and carer, as part of his or her pastoral caring, must be a strong advocate for education, challenging and correcting any misinformation on the subject of the disease. It is important to challenge all blaming, all scapegoating and all discriminatory treatment of those infected with the virus and those associated with them. But this can only occur if we have courage and integrity of purpose, thus enabling us to be fearlessly affirmative in our standing alongside the infected person or anyone else directly affected.

In affirming pastoral care, we are involved in our common vulnerability and frailty, with all its strengths and weaknesses. The extent of our fearfulness mirrors our own inability to

* In Victor Gong and Norman Rudnick (Eds), *AIDS: facts and issues* (Rutgers University Press, 1986).

cope with any disease which may be infective physically, mentally and socially. We are expected to care pastorally for the PLW-HIV and those who suffer with him or her as we would any other person being debilitated by any disease.

Fear is akin to a contagious disease. It is nourished through ignorance. In listening to men and women who are suffering this viral infection, I hear these fears and anxieties:

- of losing their partners, families, friends and colleagues, through the fear of sexual contact, of being infected and of infecting others
- of rejection, of humiliation and violence, including the violence of bigotry and the 'Wrath of God' pronouncements
- of scapegoating, the blaming of gays and drug addicts for the so-called 'plague', by some irresponsible media
- of losing jobs and promotion prospects, of losing accommodation and mortgage possibilities
- of being denied medical and dental treatment and life insurance facilities

These fears result in anxiety and depression, a kind of lostness, and can be expressed outwardly as anger against others or inwardly against self; contemplation of suicide is not uncommon and occasionally carried out.

Equally, I hear the fears and anxieties being expressed by gay groups:

- of losing equal opportunity rights
- of the closing down of all gay venues and being denied use of, and access to, public facilities, and isolation from the rest of society
- of losing funding for all gay volunteer community groups and projects
- of setback in the age of comparative consent
- of political backlash
- of increased police harassment
- of being leperised through either the use or misuse of new, or even past, legislation

Any person infected with this virus, and those associated with them, will share similar fears and anxieties whatever the mode or source of infection. While the disease is devastating

17

for all concerned, it can stimulate a tremendous drive to find a personal cure, even a religious-like conversion to the ideas of different alternative treatments.

It is increasingly the function of ministers and other carers to challenge the AFRAIDS epidemic through teaching via the homily or the sermon, through positive pastoral care and public advocacy, and through daring to be compassionately vulnerable.

This function can be achieved by attempting to understand the fears of both the infected person and of the 'worried well'. The fears of the infected person, while quite understandable, are not acceptable in those who are involved in pastoral care. Such care is not only for the well, but also the weak, the lame and especially the outcasts of society. Only by daring to allow the PLW-HIV 'to be' alongside us will we be educated into seeing, hearing and being with the real person hidden within the fears, the anxieties:

- the pain of this disease
- the pain of being rejected by partner, family, friends and a fearful society
- the fear of being disabled and disfigured physically
- the fear of losing control of one's mind, of one's life
- the additional pain in many cases of being a member of a minority whose needs and emotional nature are regarded with suspicion
- the fear of it being known that you are gradually dying from a viral infection that, for the most part, is sexually transmitted and then blood-borne to all parts of the body, especially the immune system, the protective system that in any other situation would destroy the invader rather than allow it to build up in the body – a kind of viral time-bomb.

We will only be able to meet with homosexual or bisexual men and women fully if we have come to terms with our own sexuality. To achieve this we need to be as knowledgeable as possible about our own areas of sexual anxiety and fear. Such awareness is especially important in the pastoral care of PLW-HIV and those with AIDS, as the virus is usually transmitted via sexual encounter and is no respecter of one's sexual orientation. This means that ministers and other carers must be aware of their sexual orientation and be content about it. Unless we are comfortable in our own sexual nature, we will certainly not be with those whose sexual orientation differs from our own. Only through a truthful acceptance of our own place within the sexual spectrum will we be able to offer pastoral care of a non-judgemental or non-moralising nature.

We need to remind ourselves that 'all human sexual encounters – even the most disordered, the most fleeting and possibly the most violent – involve a quest for warmth and intimacy. The needle is a symbol of ecstasy, the organism of blood. Priests who minister in this area need more, not less, warmth. But this raises the question about how at ease we are with our own sexuality and about our own willingness to give and receive affection.'* It is crucial to all pastoral care that we realise that everyone especially Christians must search out the meaning of the gift of sexuality that may, or may not, have an overt sexual expression. The Church, like so many individuals (professional and otherwise), is being called on a pilgrimage into the mysteries of the gift of sexuality and of its co-creative and/or co-destructive potential.

Being accepting, open and fearless of our own specific orientation allows us to approach and embrace others with a gentle, quiet, non-condemning compassion. Through such an embrace, we will recognise and accept the uniqueness, the utter humanness of the PLW-HIV sufferer and those who suffer alongside him or her.

This fear of sexuality is often accompanied by the fear of touching a person whose sexual orientation differs from our own. For this reason, some ministers and other carers are unable to embrace the sufferer who is attempting to live with the virus and its unknown activity within the body. This is because many people are quite ignorant of the ways in which the virus can be communicated. We simply *cannot* be infected through the touch of embracing.

This point has been demonstrated clearly to us by the Archbishop of Canterbury in his lengthy visit to a hospital in

* Unpublished paper by Kenneth Leech, 'The AIDS Crisis and Pastoral Care – some wider issues', a talk given at a conference on AIDS, Nashotah House, Wisconsin, USA, 4 April 1986.

December 1986. Since then HRH the Princess of Wales and Norman Fowler, then Minister of Health, have made similar visits. Nurses and doctors would not bring their very young children into such wards if there were the slightest possibility of contracting the virus other than by the known routes of infection.

It is therefore the pastoral responsibility of every minister, every carer, whether professional or voluntary, to use their specific pastoral gifts to communicate this message. It is no good evading the issue in order to avoid offending others. Besides, a lively and sensitive awareness will, in most instances, prevent such offence occurring.

Fear, I believe, can be classed as a communicable disease, perhaps more virulent than the viral infection itself. Therefore, we must be especially vigilant to see that we do not communicate fear instead of hope. It is our loving that will cast out all fear.

Those infected with the virus will often experience one or all of the following:

- shock of diagnosis and having to face death early in one's life
- feeling of powerlessness to change circumstances, and consequent frustration and anger
- reduced physical functioning because of declining health
- anxiety about the reactions of others, with consequent social withdrawal and loss of social support
- reduced cognitive functioning because of anxiety, depression, obsessional worries, and possible intellectual impairment
- reduced sexual functioning, loss of libido and erectile dysfunction
- fear of infecting others, particularly partners
- concern about the partner and how he, or she, will cope
- fear of being deserted and of dying alone
- fear of dying in pain and discomfort
- social, domestic and occupational disruption

The following is a brief list of the fears and anxieties often expressed by partners, families and friends of those infected:

- fear about the possible death of the partner, grief, shock and sense of helplessness
- fear of being infected, leading to anxiety, depression and obsessional worries
- reduced sexual functioning, especially loss of libido and loss of prospect of future sex
- guilt about the possibility of having infected the partner and others
- uncertainty about what to do next – conflict between avoiding infection and the need to express physical love of one's partner arouses guilt and can lead to psychological, cognitive and emotional confusion
- uncertainty about what to do to help the partner
- clinical anxiety and depression

We need to be aware of the problems of those who know themselves to be 'body positive', i.e. living with HIV infection, and who are fearful of developing the 'Full-blown AIDS' syndrome. They may experience:

- anxiety about having AIDS or the virus
- depression about the perceived inevitability of infection, and/or developing the full syndrome
- morbid obsession about the disease with constant checking for symptoms
- guilt about being homosexual and the resurrection of past 'misdemeanours'
- social, domestic and occupational disruption and stress during their illness

It is the responsibility of the pastoral carers to help the infected person to adjust to what is happening on a day-by-day basis and yet to remain positively strong in his or her attitudes. There is a great deal of growing evidence that affirming a person's self-image and continuing value is a real way of helping the immune system to continue to resist the full development of the AIDS syndrome.

Support can be offered by:

- maintaining a truthful, but hopeful, attitude in all stages of the illness
- taking time simply to be with the person on his or her

terms, and not being put off if after making the journey to see the person one is then asked within five minutes to leave
- taking in news and letters that will keep the person in touch with the community
- taking in small tokens of friendship, for instance, a flower, cigarettes, sweets, a pizza, fruit or fruit juice
- taking the person out for a walk or drive if possible, or out to a meal – change of scenery is so important
- sharing in any discussions the person may initiate
- being sensitive to the strain or non-strain of your visit – frequent short visits are preferable to an occasional long visit
- quietly sharing in the needs of his or her partner and family
- perhaps the most difficult work is simply to remain quietly alongside, letting the *silence* speak of our mutual pain, our mutual love.

Only love will cast out all fears – love of the kind that ennobles and authenticates those in the depths of the viral infection, affirming their uniqueness, their worth that is beyond all costing.

4

In the Pain

I became involved in the pastoral care of AIDS sufferers early in 1985, when I volunteered my services to the Terrence Higgins Trust. The Trust was the first group of people to be expressly concerned with this growing area of need, and it now provides a considerable number of services for persons living with the new viral infection and those caring for them, i.e. their partners, families, friends and colleagues.

The pain shared often begins with the person coming for advice as to whether or not he should take the test, or when he informs us that he has AIDS, although he probably means he is antibody positive.

If he is seeking advice on whether or not to take the test, there should be a general discussion as to why he feels he should and the pros and cons for taking the test. Should he then decide to do so (see p. 90), it is important that he should be involved in pre- and post-testing counselling with a knowledgeable member of the Sexually Transmitted Disease clinic (STD), usually the doctor, health adviser and/or nurse. Unless the minister or other carer knows the facts about the new viral infection, it is better simply to be alongside the person, as you would anyone anticipating a test which will have a devastating effect on him or her if found to be positive.

At this stage the person does not have AIDS. The test only suggests that he has been infected at some time within the past three to seven years, depending on the type of virus. The test is not absolutely perfect and the person, once tested, should be voluntarily re-tested at three-monthly intervals, especially if remaining sexually active.

Whether the person receives a negative or positive test result, it is extremely prudent that he practices safer sex.

23

Although there are epidemiological reasons for encouraging the taking of the test, no one should be pressurised into doing so, because almost unbearable personal anxiety and stress will follow, including a further depression of the immune system that may well be under pressure already from the possible viral infection.

When someone informs us that he has AIDS, we need to enquire gently when, where and by whom he was informed – whether by telephone, letter, his general practitioner, a non-medical person, or a member of a Sexually Transmitted Disease clinic.

The shock of being informed that one is HIV positive can be lessened or enhanced by *how* one is informed. As an illustration of this, I quote with the author's full permission an experience from *inside* the situation, far better expressed than I, from *outside*, could ever do.

The diagnosis

It was Friday the 11th July 1986 at half past one in the afternoon when I found out that I had the virus . . .

Despite my awareness of the possibilities, I was not in the least prepared for the news. Though outwardly calm, I went into instant shock. I recall the doctor gently telling me through a dark cloud that I also had a severe case of herpes, a fungal infection, pneumonia and that I should have to be admitted on the spot. I had great difficulty following what he was saying for each word he spoke became immediately transformed into that word, 'DEATH!' I was aware of the duality of what he was saying and of what echoed within. Confusion rebounded in my head till it hurt and I wanted to run like hell. This wasn't happening to me. I don't want it. I damn well refuse to own this disease. There must be some mistake. I heard myself refuse point blank to be admitted. Was he not, after all, telling me to come in to die? How dare he! The more gently insistent he became the more aggressively defensive I heard myself responding. I was shocked at my own behaviour. Another doctor was brought and I was given a complete physical examination. I found the doctor's touch

24

gave me great comfort. In the end, I was allowed home with massive doses of antibiotics and on the understanding that I would return at the slightest sign of the pneumonia worsening. I remained in that state of deep shock for the remainder of the day, taking taxis from one tea room to another, leaving £5 tips wherever I went. It proved to be a most expensive day!

Death and dying

All the ills passed as the antibiotics did their work over the next couple of weeks but for months afterwards I became completely preoccupied with thoughts of death. My death. I so wanted to talk about death in general and my death in particular but people, otherwise kind caring people, refused to allow me to do so. An irritating pattern began to emerge. I would talk about the very real possibility of going on to develop 'Full-blown AIDS' and of the known outcome, death. My friends, not hearing the meaning behind what I was saying, would invariably counter with, 'Well you could get knocked down in the road tomorrow.' Or, 'Death comes to us all at some time.' I knew they were trying to comfort me but these comments only left me feeling angry. They too wanted to run like hell and make believe that it wasn't true and I had to fight to get them to listen to what concerned me. With many, I gave up quite quickly as an act of compassion for *they* suffered in attempting to talk about my possible death. Besides, we didn't have a shared language to help us get to the heart of the meaning.

Rejection, self-rejection and the strength to be alone

I would much prefer the comfort of religious faith but I have none. Not even to blame. I am utterly alone . . .

In an attempt to find someone to talk to about my state of shock, my illness and possible death, I contacted a well-known psychotherapy centre and one at which I was known and where I had been a long standing client. They refused even to see me. I was frankly amazed, but felt the positive potential of anger rise within me at this rejection and in defence of selfhood. The fighting spirit at least was alive and well. Courage was becoming more important by the day.

Courage, however, was not always available when it was needed. I found myself becoming depressed and more than once thoughts of suicide – a chance to decide – came to me, thoughts I was ashamed of and felt I couldn't share with others – not least because I constantly reminded myself that, had I not been gay, then this would never have happened. Perhaps those 'Jesus freaks' were right and this was the result of a wasted life. Thoughts like these, and others far more extreme, came and went. I was becoming scared of cracking up completely. I knew that the growing depression was anger turned inwards towards self but, despite the intellectual awareness, I was unable to do anything about it. I began to hate myself and everything gay.

At a point of an all-time low, I telephoned a friend who is well versed in the issues of AIDS to seek his advice and within minutes found myself crying. I'd never cried like this. My whole body was involved. I hurt all over. He came to my home and the first thing he said was, 'I've no intention of counselling you.' Instead, he put his arms around me and stroked me. I burst into tears and cried and shouted for four hours. He never let go. I attempted to move away but he saw the meaning and held and stroked me even more tenderly. I was glad to have such a friend. Afterwards we talked. He let me talk through all my crazy and not so crazy thoughts. All the anger and pain came flooding out and so too did the depression. It has not troubled me since. When he left hours later, I felt safe with myself. The telephone had been so useful. It allowed me to test out a possible rejection without having to find out face to face. Having discovered this once, I used the same method with others. It's simple and it helped.

Discovering laughter again
One such friend listened to how I felt like a leper and how I'd thought of getting myself a bell to ring. She listened. When I stopped, she offered advice on the kind of bell that might be right for me. I seem to recall that she discounted

26

church bells as being too heavy and settled on a bicycle bell. Within minutes, she had me laughing at myself. It was a good feeling. Through humour and laughter, I saw how crazy were my thoughts. She laughed with me and, in so doing, I knew instinctively that she wasn't laughing at me. Sure my thoughts were becoming morbid but they were also quite funny too.

Consequences

I watched an American television production with my closest friend. It was called *Buddies* and was about a young man dying of AIDS and another young man who came to befriend him. (This television movie can teach you far more than I can about what a person needs who has AIDS – I have a copy.) Anyway, there was a scene when the buddie asks the AIDS patient what he would do if he had just one healthy day. I found myself in quite a state as my mind played with the notion. I guess what I was feeling was grief for my mind played the same scene over and over again. I was kissing and hugging all my nephews and nieces. I know that I will never again kiss another person on the lips and the knowledge of that hurts so much . . .

Despite the great need I have to be held and loved, I still feel scared when someone hugs me or kisses my cheeks. The bottom line is that I don't want to contaminate them. I still often feel dirty and to blame. Intellectually, I have enough knowledge to realise that there is absolutely no reason in the world to stop kissing just as I realise that I am not to blame for having the virus. But my emotions twist and distort the logical and rational into a shape which reflects the virus itself. When I pull back from a hug or a kiss, it is myself I'm pulling away from, not you.

I'm capable of becoming almost completely paranoid at the slightest sign of infection in others. I don't mean those with the virus. I mean those with the common cold, those with a slight cough and those with throat infections. I'm so aware that my immune defence system is at risk and that I may not be able physically to deal with the next sneeze. I sometimes just want to shut myself away from everyone and, from time to time, I do just that. When I've done so, however, I became so lonely that I now try, often with great effort, to keep up social contacts.

What does an AIDS sufferer require?
This is my own personal check list of twenty:
- support when considering taking the test
- the facts about the test and its outcome
- updated information about the nature of AIDS
- a friend to go with me when I get the results (I went alone)
- time to absorb emotionally the results with the doctor (I was given none)
- a short paper to explain the results (I was given nothing)
- counselling or psychotherapy (I was refused by a therapist)
- a private space to retreat
- an opportunity to shout, cry, curse, blame, demand answers, talk about whatever comes, plan one's death, write a will, choose a doctor, feel, talk of suicide, be shocking, be illogical, laugh, be confused, change, find a meaning, and react spontaneously
- frank open talking about the virus
- respect
- courage
- a chance to help others
- a reason to go on living
- contact with others
- sex (I choose solo activity)
- understanding from others about fatigue
- a washing machine to cope with sheets drenched with night sweats
- regular food, breaks, exercise, sleep
- truth about one's condition

In the main, I've come to terms with having the virus but find that the unexpected emotion can change things overnight. My own personal response is to attempt to give purpose to all that I do. *More than ever before, I find myself* *working upon improving the quality of my life and less upon thinking about the quantity.**

AIDS

It's all daggers, knives and blades!
When friend becomes foe,
You know how they go,
When you mention that you've got AIDS!

So declare it, hear it, wear it!
When you die so do I.
I have tears when you cry.
Oh, how, in your name, do you bear it?

I'm tempted, like some, to hide,
Quietly, my energy save,
Gladly go to my grave,
And be buried along with my pride.

But I'm angry, I'll shout and I'll write.
I reject all blame,
Don't enter that game,
It's *people* who die, so fight!

Every action produces another,
It's Gays, in the main,
Who carry the pain,
So stand alongside your brother.

RICHIE J. MCMULLEN

* Richie McMullen, *Living with HIV in self and others* (Gay Men's Press, 1988).

5

Sharing the Pain

*The least you offer to one of these my brothers
and sisters you offer to me*

During the latter half of 1985, I was asked by Tony Whitehead of the Terrence Higgins Trust if I would visit a very ill
man who was suffering from 'Full-blown AIDS'. He had
expressed the desire to see a priest – 'the one who goes into
the pubs in the Earls Court area'. I am the priest he was
looking for and, without hesitation, I said I would visit Tom
that same day.

Tom

Tom,* in his own unique way, taught me about the good and
the bad aspects of being severely ill with AIDS and the havoc
it can create for all concerned. I arrived and found him to be
a very fine-looking young man of about twenty-five, who
appeared to be in reasonably good health. However, his
appearance belied what was actually going on inside his body,
which was limp with exhaustion after any excessive movement. His anxiety about this was very evident.

Tom had been living for about five years in the USA and
with his partner for the past three years. Tom was an artist
and his partner an actor (a few years older than him). About
a year prior to returning to England, Tom had been diagnosed
antibody positive, yet he had remained reasonably healthy
for a further nine months. After a month in England, staying

---

* The names of those who allowed me to be alongside them and their
situations have been changed.

with two very close friends (Richard and Michael), it was quite evident that Tom needed hospital treatment. A doctor was called and his admission arranged.

Richard and Michael continued to look after Tom. They visited him daily and made phone calls to his partner in America. Tom flatly refused to have his father notified that he was seriously ill in hospital. He often said, 'My father would never understand. We have never really been close.' During my frequent visits to Tom, he expressed many anxieties, principally that his family would find out that he was a homosexual and that he had a 'lover' who meant more to him than anyone else in his life except his mother. He was anxious about dying, but more so about *how* he would die. Would he meet up with his mother who had died of cancer three months previously? Would she be annoyed because he could not attend her funeral? 'If there is a God, will he punish me for being queer? I would like to believe that God and my mother will love me always.'

During the first month of his stay in hospital, it seemed to me that Tom decided to let go of his life. 'There is no future here for me that is worth having.' He asked that his partner be telephoned in America to say that he wished to see him. Tom also asked that his father and his aunt should visit him, but without being told why he was ill. He wished them to be told simply that he was seriously ill with pneumonia which, in a sense, was true. These requests were met through Richard and Michael. Colin arrived from America within twenty-four hours and was at Tom's bedside when Tom's father and aunt arrived. His father, on arriving and finding his son not only seriously ill but in the arms of his partner, was infuriated and ordered the 'lover' out of the room. An argument ensued and, finally, Colin gave way.

I could feel the anger and the pain for the immediate trio. The father, on being informed of the true nature of his son's illness, found out for the first time that he was homosexual, and dying. This, coupled with the loss of his wife three months before, was a heavy load to carry. The partner was antagonistic towards the father, knowing he had never had much time for his son, and resented his attitude towards Tom now that he was dying. The father was devastated because his son was dying of (for him) an unacceptable disease which Colin might have given him, despite all Colin's tests having proved negative. Here was a pain that was beyond words and could somehow only be embraced in the silence of trying to be with them both in the uniqueness of their individual pain.

Tom died about a week after seeing his father and Colin. I felt at the time, and still do, that he had decided to make his exit and on his own terms. Unfortunately, the partner and father had great difficulty in being in the same room together. The situation was defused to some extent by Richard and Michael, who took it in turns to be there with them. So, his two special friends helped to ease and to carry the pain, alongside their own pain. Tom's partner and father were quite unable to share each other's pain although I personally found it difficult to see how their love for Tom could not help them to do so.

The friends arranged the funeral service which I was asked to lead. I was fearful of what might occur as, when Tom died, his father was so full of pain that he suggested his son's body should be thrown away. I spent considerable time with Tom's father and Colin, who were both quite adamant that, if the other turned up at the funeral, they would leave. Both, as it happened, did attend the service without acknowledging each other and left in different directions afterwards.

Spending some time with Tom's father after the service, I felt that he was a little less angry but I was proved wrong. When his son's ashes were to be picked up and placed in his mother's grave, the father ordered the crematorium to throw the ashes away and not to tell anyone where. I often think of this father and hope the wounds will eventually be healed and that he will recognise the innate goodness in his son. Colin contacted me the day after the funeral and asked for one thing – a copy of my homily as he could not take much of it in at the service itself. At his request, I typed it out and handed it to him with a large card that had a butterfly on its cover, a symbol of new life.

Barry

Barry, the youngest person I have attempted to minister to, was a young man suffering from Kaposi's sarcoma, a form of cancer involving not only the skin but also the internal organs of the body. At fifteen, Barry 'came out' to his parents as being homosexual and at twenty-one (when I met him) had been sharing his life with another man in a monogamous relationship for three years. Trevor (his partner) was about twenty-four. It was obvious that they were devoted to each other and each family felt that it had gained another son. Both men were quite popular and genuinely loved by their parents. Barry was hardly ever without a visitor. As he became increasingly weaker and more aware of his dying, he became more and more consoling to Trevor – 'my mate' – and their respective parents. Whether Barry or Trevor ever went to church is debatable. However, both believed in what they called 'the mystery'.

About two days before he died, Barry asked me, and the others round his bed, to 'think of me going on a voyage and that my bags are packed for the greatest trip ever. My passport has been approved and I am simply waiting for the plane to take off into the mystery.' He added that when he got to his destination, he would wait for us. Barry had clearly gone through all the stages of letting go and he was now, simply, waiting for the journey to begin.

I was not with Barry when he died. However, my last picture was of him surrounded by those he dearly loved and who dearly loved him. His mother was holding his left hand, his partner was holding his right hand, and his father was embracing them all. This, for me, was a real live symbol of 'Our Father' who embraces and enfolds us all within the love of understanding acceptance.

Robert

Robert was admitted to hospital suffering from a form of pneumocystis carinii. As well as the physical disease he was suffering from extreme anxiety about his wife and son. He was also deeply guilty for putting Joan through so much anguish. During their marriage he had had occasional sexual involvements with men and somewhere became infected with the HIV virus. His wife was very supportive but was herself not being supported by either his or her family and she had to carry the burden alone. She was fearful of approaching her local parish priest. 'I know he would not understand.' When I held her in my arms, I could feel her pain as together we tried to share and prepare for the inevitable. Robert, who adored his son, could hardly look at him when he visited with his mother. Kenny thought coming to London was great; he was too young to understand fully the 'why' of Daddy's illness.

During his time in hospital, Robert would share his thoughts with me, principally of the pain his wife was enduring because their respective families had made lepers of them. His was not a 'hopeful' dying. He could not feel he was being made ready to be received by his creator, and I am not sure that I enabled him to feel he was indeed being loved by our ultimate lover, God our Father, who understood (as no other) the creative potential of our falling short of the mark of perfection. All I am aware of is that, as a member of the caring team, there was little I could do except to be with him, his wife and his son, trusting that, in some way, Robert was being healed, integrated into the ultimate mystery of being alive to all life in the here and now of his dying to the life for which he had been born.

Fred

The following story shows how co-creative, co-healing potential can be shared within the depths of a disease that appears to offer no hope.

During the past year, I was asked to see Fred, a man of about thirty-five, dying as a result of repeated attacks of opportunistic infections with which his severely damaged immune system was unable to cope. His doctor said to me: 'Father Bill, I feel he is searching and you may be able to help him.' I responded by going to Fred's room, but immediately he saw my collar he said: 'I'm an atheist and I don't

34

want you or any other churchy person.' I respected this and quietly walked out of his room.

A couple of days later he saw me walking past his room and asked: 'What's wrong with me? Don't I rate a visit?' I responded immediately and sat beside him for about fifteen minutes, neither of us saying anything.

Suddenly, the floodgates opened with a barrage of questions like: 'Do you really think I'm a sinner because I'm gay?'

I replied with something along these lines: 'I have not given it a thought as, up to now, we have not spoken. I do not know where you are coming from and, therefore, it would be wrong for me to judge you. But, now that you mention it, I feel we all fall short of the mark of perfection and, in this, we can all be labelled sinners. However, for me, the greatest sin is not to love or allow ourselves to be loved.'

'Well, Bill,' he said, 'I have loved the same man for twenty-five years. Doesn't that count for something?'

I replied, 'Truthful love counts for everything. For me, to be in love is to be in God who is within every person he created and knows to be good. For me the mystery of God is the mystery of love and that love never ever casts out love. Similarly, I believe that love is able to understand and to cope with all our unloving ways to which we are all vulnerable.'

After a very long silence between us, holding hands, he said, 'I love my partner and that is all I can leave him. Is that enough?'

I could only reply, 'What greater gift could you leave him?'

After another long space of silence, he took my hand to his chest and said, 'You are not a priest, you are a lover.' I simply replied that I hoped they were one and the same.

During this time of in-depth sharing according to Fred's wish, something rich opened up for both of us – a kind of unlocking of the channels for our mutual healing. Just as I was leaving, his partner walked in to continue his vigil and to encourage Fred that it was all right to leave him now for they would always be together with the gift of their mutual loving.

For me, this was a moving experience – I would dare to call it a mystical experience – shared. Fred died in Jonathan's arms during the next twenty-four hours and all agreed he had a fine transition into the next dimension of his journey into the life that awaits us all. Surely all we can say when we are so privileged is 'Thanks be to God. *Thanks be to Love.*'

Being involved in shared caring – potentially the most co-creative human endeavour – I have come to feel with an inner knowing that HIV infection must be viewed as a challenge and as an opportunity for a compassion that ennobles the sufferer. As the receiver and the offerer, we can allow a mutuality of service to develop as we cry out with those in pain. Linked as we are with the enforced lonely ones, weak as we are with the weak, vulnerable with the vulnerable, powerless with the powerless, we are strengthened by the mutuality of care with, and for, each other. We need to be compassionate, to go where it hurts, to enter into places of pain and to share in the anguish of an unknown path through the various opportunistic infections.

If we are to be faithful to the continuing pastorship of Jesus, we should behave as he behaved towards sufferers of every kind, especially those branded as lepers. Through his example, we have no choice but to embrace all those infected with the HIV virus and those who suffer with them. This is the work of God in Christ and of Christ in us. It is also the work of love's compassionate endeavouring towards *all* who suffer. Every minister should be aware of the need to be humble enough to allow the sufferer to minister to him or to her, as they surely do, through their own unique ways of suffering. It is the mystery of *our shared pain* that releases the mutuality of our compassion. If one member of the human family suffers, all suffer. If one member is infected with the HIV virus, all are infected. To the extent that one member of the Body of Christ is infected, then the Body of the Church is also infected.

I would like us to picture an image of Christ suffering with HIV infection and remind ourselves of what Hans Küng wrote about Christ's first followers. His description could well apply to those moving through the different stages of HIV infection:

This people, a flock without a shepherd, feeling misunderstood by both the establishment and the rebels, despised by the pharasaical devout individuals of the towns and villages and by the ascetics of the desert, useless for either temple or military service, incapable of exact observance of the law and still less of major ascetic achievement; this is the people on whom Jesus has compassion – these who are called blessed, who are not enfranchised, who can be neglected and abused with impunity at all times by the ruling parties and authorities, these must feel he understands them. They are for him.*

The main issue of this infection for the minister and other carers is whether or not we are prepared to offer *unconditional* compassion as an expression, not only of our own love, but also of the love of God in us.

Our caring, as best we are able, for individuals who are suffering from various stages of HIV infection, does not have to be justified in any way, but *any lack of compassionate caring on our part certainly does need justification.*

I hope our pastoral caring will be such that all those in our concern will feel and know we care about them at all times, in all places and at every level of infection. Compassion demands the total presence of the minister within the unlimited embrace of acceptance and hope, nourished as it is by the love of God in Christ and Christ in each other. It is through our pastoral caring, shared with others, that we shall enable the sufferer and those who share the suffering to know:

God loves us, as love loving us.

God embraces us, as love embracing us.

God reaches out to us, as love reaching out to us
    through the frailties that are our common bond.

I have tried to be as objective as I can in relating my experiences with Tom, Barry, Robert and Fred in order to illustrate what might seem impossible: that each and every person has his or her own unique perception of the mystery of God – for many the 'unnameable'. I have also tried to show the vast differences that the minister and others involved in pastoral caring must be prepared to meet when offering

* Hans Küng, *On Being a Christian* (Collins, 1977).

such a vulnerable ministry towards those who themselves could not be more vulnerable to the viral infection and the opportunistic infections.

As a vulnerable minister, I come away from each situation with different feelings but essentially feelings of anger at my apparent helplessness to heal some of the damage done to those whose life styles both individuals and the Church have difficulty in recognising as being co-creative in their potential. I sometimes come away impatient with my inability simply to be with the person in so far as this is possible, remembering of course that I am not the person with the infection and all its ramifications. All of this is enhanced by the fact that most of those we are ministering to are between the ages of twenty-one and forty, the young-middle generation of men and women now being deprived of their future. It is particularly painful to watch a young person's body disintegrate or his or her frequent loss of memory.

The emotional strain can, at times, be very heavy indeed. More than once have I cried into a friend's shoulder, while being held very close, with the pain of it all. You find yourself crying for those who are unable to cry; you cry after the manner that Christ did as he cried out from the cross for the pain of all humankind, past, present and future. The echo of this cry of pain is of feeling lost in what so often appears to be a vast sea of hopelessness, as the viral infection takes over the whole person, who desperately needs to be authenticated into an understanding of their own innate goodness.

As a minister, it is so easy to become a father-figure, because the distance between the sufferer and the person offering pastoral care is full of need at a level I have never previously experienced in other areas of nursing and pastoral caring. I find myself being a father-figure both for my own needs and also for the needs of the person, just as a father would take the hand of a suffering son or daughter and, like a father, find no difficulty in 'kissing it better'. One learns as a father or mother the healing value of touch, of being held, especially in those situations where there are no answers.

I also know how vital it is for ministers to keep what could be called a 'healing distance', and I constantly learn through those to whom I am attempting to offer pastoral care how not to become too personally involved. It is important that I maintain the space that is so essential not only for the person in need of care but, equally, for the person offering care.

This space is essential, because of the strength of the emotional involvement with each person. I myself feel it is essential for each minister or other carer to have a 'spiritual director' – a soul friend or an enabling comrade – and be linked into supportive therapy, either in an individual situation or within a group which is aware of the pressures of this kind of ministry. It must be a group in which one feels safe and in which there is much trust and confidentiality. It must be a group in which one can allow oneself to be cared for in order that one may be all the more present to those with whom one is in contact. It is this group, or that special person whom one trusts, who will constantly remind one of one's frailties and one's potential for 'burn-out', which can so easily happen in this particular area of care.

It is crucial for the minister and all others offering pastoral care to remember that there are others quite as capable, if not more so, of sharing in this ministry and that all forms of ministry, of pastoral care, begin with pastoral care towards oneself, simply because it is through oneself (in association with others including those living with HIV infection and those who suffer with them) that really meaningful pastoral care takes place. Together we remember that we are all wounded enablers of healing and that pastoral care is a shared activity of the Church. It is a vital function of the Church to show concern for each and every person as we proclaim, in and through our actions, that we are indeed following in the steps of Jesus. Together we travel the uniqueness of our inner/outer journeys towards the wholeness of the person we are endeavouring to become.

To be a minister or carer is to be a lover, not only of others, but also of oneself. In this way, we are held together in the ministry through the workings of the 'ultimate lover', our Father, who is also our mother, who can do no other than embrace all they created and know to be intrinsically good. As God has faith in us, so he has a hope for us, as he embraces us with love, that we too might grow in faith, hope and love, not only for those who are our pastoral concern at any one time but also for ourselves.

It is this that we are to offer: the ministry that is above all ministries, that of *love*.

Morning Call

'Morning Call', taken from a prayer card,* invites us to join each other, whenever possible, at 8 o'clock each morning in reciting a familiar prayer such as Our Father, Hail Mary, Glory Be or the Jesus prayer, or devoting a period of silence, on behalf of:

• all those infected with HIV, to whatever degree; for their physical, mental and spiritual health; for those who love them; and especially for those who have no one to pray for them
• all who minister, in whatever capacity, to those who suffer from the effects of HIV infection
• those engaged in research: that a vaccine against the virus and a cure for AIDS may be speedily found
• the success of Health Education Schemes: that they may halt the spread of HIV
• the souls of those who have died of AIDS, and especially for those who have died estranged from the ministrations of the Church, and for those who had no one to pray for them.

Here are two prayers from the same source which I find helpful:

Dear Lord,
    You entered into the world and became flesh so that the love that abides with the world still could be seen and felt. By your grace, enable me to enter into your healing life with loving and caring action as your spirit shall lead. Amen.

* Published by Christian Action on AIDS, 1987, and obtainable from PO Box 76, Hereford HR1 1JX.

Dear Lord,

You came into the world so that we should know your love and care for us. By your grace help me to share your loving and caring with those whose lives are being changed by the AIDS virus and to bring them help and comfort. Amen.

6

Death and Bereavement

Death always has been and always will be with us. It is an integral part of human existence. And because it is, it has always been a subject of deep concern to all of us. Since the dawn of humankind, the human mind has pondered death, searching for the answer to its mysteries. For the key to the question of death unlocks the door to life.

*It is by dying that we flow into the final stages of a growth that is unique to each and every person.**

Dying into the completeness of life

When people come to us for pastoral care, whether they be PLW-HIV, partners, relatives or friends, it is really essential to help them cope with their own very strong feelings of anger, sorrow, failure or guilt, some of which will be buried very deeply in their subconscious. They may deny what is really happening or be bargaining for the person's life to continue. They may be in the deep depression of preparatory grief or have begun to accept the prognosis and be trying to live on the very difficult day-to-day process.

For the practising Christian, the Church's traditional ministries of healing and reconciliation may be of some support. For the non-Christian, however, the laying-on-of-hands or the touch of an embrace is also very comforting, especially in the terminal stages of the infection when AIDS sufferers feel themselves to be the modern lepers, the untouchables. The touch of the embrace is the touch of acceptance: of love's compassion.

* Elisabeth Kübler-Ross, *Death, the Final Stage of Growth* (Simon & Schuster, 1986).

Bearing in mind that we will be stretched to the limits of our personal resources as we attempt to respond with the compassion of care, we have to remember that, as the person dies, our own feelings of helplessness become all the more acute. Our pastoral responsibility is to assure the sufferer of his or her continuing value as an essentially unique person reaching out and into the mystery of mysteries, awaiting the major departure in life to life.

Stages of grieving

Our grief begins from the moment we are aware of another's dying or indeed of our own. Anticipatory grief, as it is known, is a psychological reaction to impending death frequently experienced by the person who is dying and by the partner, family and other carers. It can occur during any long debilitating illness of a terminal nature. We must not forget that the dying are more often than not intent upon mourning *their own* passing as we, indeed, are preparing to mourn theirs.

Neither must we forget that in instances of sudden death (and these do occur with those who are suffering from severe HIV infection) comfort is needed long after most comforters have ceased giving it. Flashbacks are common in all grieving, particularly at birthdays, Christmas and other special anniversaries.

To be aware of the different stages of bereavement in others, we need to recognise our own personal involvement in it. Will our concern have any effect on the person who is going through the process? We need to be aware of where, and how, the bereavement touches us.

There are seven possible stages of the grieving process, a process which is so essential if we are to be integrated and re-established in a fullness of life that is worth both living and dying for.

The *first stage* is usually *shock*. On hearing of the death of a loved partner or member of the family or friend, all expectations are shattered. Shock is often followed by denial or disbelief. Everything is saying 'no' to death.

Words are of no real comfort at this time. Comfort comes from the quiet presence of someone who cares, keeping the

43

griever in touch with life. The grieving person at this time will do one of two things: either withdraw into self or explode verbally, perhaps even use physical violence – usually towards inanimate objects, but also towards self.

We are shocked and confused by the tragedy of a young person's death just as we are angry and confused by the death of a child. Such young deaths deprive them, and us, of the potential that was theirs, and ours through them.

The *second stage* in the dynamics of grief is that of *disorganisation*. This can take various forms from being out of touch with everyday, ordinary activities through to confusion which is the normal manifestation. In such cases, the principal need is the constant physical presence of a person whom the griever knows and can trust. Grievers need physical contact that is both warm and embracing, a presence in which they are able to cry and cry, to talk and talk without interruptions. The pain needs to flow out. No decisions should be made by the person at this time.

In the *third stage*, the bereaved person will release very *heavy emotions* through being made to feel safe in the embracing presence of someone who will not fade away out of fear, as the bereaved person expresses feelings of helplessness, hurt, frustration, of being abandoned. Unless the griever feels safe to explode outwards, then it will take place internally and could lead to very serious physical and mental disturbances. The release comes through the gift of permissive listening. Through such listening, the bereaved person learns that such feelings are neither good nor bad. They are *there* to be released.

In the *fourth stage*, feelings of *guilt* beset the bereaved person whose loving relationship has been shattered by death. Unfortunately, the guilt-prone mourner will find abundant reasons to intensify his or her guilt. There seems to be a need to punish oneself. We have to be careful in this stage, as with any other. What may be being intensified at this time is lifelong guilt that the mourner may be harbouring. Patient and permissive listening is the key to this situation. So much of what sound like cries of guilt are only loud and testing pleas for assurance that there is nothing to feel guilty about.

At the *fifth stage*, there is a great sense of loss and loneliness, perhaps the most painful time. The loss and resultant loneliness are often felt many months after support is thought necessary. As the sense of loss grows, sadness and depression feed self-pity. During this period, the person who feels lost can become difficult and the person who has died becomes a saint. This is because the grieving heart needs to have the void filled with a comforter. Friends in the pub can be closer than lifelong friends who are far away.

At this time, the frequent and regular presence of a stabilising friend becomes essential and, in fact, is essential even if only temporary. Dogs and cats can ease this pain but the real presence of another person is even more effective.

Freedom and happiness will come in the future if we can be beside the person in his or her grief in such a way that they may move to and fro through the whole process for up to two years or more. We should never push the person through or around this stage of bereavement.

At the *sixth stage* comes the feeling of relief that is so often kept bottled up. By this death, we have been freed from the many demands of love that we have had difficulty in coping with. When we are released from having to measure up to someone else's standards, we feel guilty about being freed to be ourselves for others, as well as for ourselves. All brands of relationship of love can be a mixture of love's demands and love's rewards.

These feelings of relief do not necessarily imply any criticism of the love we lost. It is instead a reflection of our need for ever deeper love which we are morally free to pursue. These feelings of relief are natural. If we do not accept this fact, we shall become burdened with unnecessary guilt. In this stage of the bereavement process, the griever needs an understanding, an enabling listener in whose presence they can express and tolerate what, at first, seems to be the most ignoble of human thoughts – relief at a loved one's death.

The *seventh stage* demonstrates that it is essential for the honesty within the grieving process to be accepted and embraced. In time, with the loving help and concern of friends and relatives, grieving persons will eventually arrive at the final stage of re-establishment of self with self and others, as increased hope softens guilt and the sense of loss. Fantasies of a new life become part of each working day, because there is now a meaning to life as one learns to walk again. Now, the phone and doorbell are answered. Invitations are accepted as firm steps replace the hesitant steps of the mourner. During this phase, old friends are important for encouragement and permission to live again.

New friends can offer realistic opportunities for coming out from under this grieving mantle. One is no longer a widow or widower. One is a person again and the yesterday of mourning is laid to rest with the beloved partner in the mystery beyond our comprehension. This movement must feel natural for the person concerned and be within his or her own timing.

These seven stages of grieving differ for each person, depending on the length of the dying process (which may begin at confirmed medical diagnosis). The time the mourner has to prepare can affect the pattern of grieving.

In the midst of all our attempts to comfort, a sense of humour is needed of the kind that will offer a realistic focus to our foibles and those in the people we love. The gift of real humour shakes up the grief of the heart so that it can be re-formed, changed if you like, through the humour of love.

Such laughter unleashes the healing power within, thus releasing the person to love themselves and even to enjoy the fact that he or she is able to love another. This is because the person for whom he or she grieves loved them and now releases them to love another and allow the other to love him or her.

A poem by Marjorie Pizer expresses for me the different ways of meeting grief:

I had thought that your death
Was a waste and a destruction,
A pain of grief hardly to be endured.
I am only beginning to learn
That your life was a gift and a growing
And a loving left with me.
The desperation of death
Destroyed the existence of love.
But the fact of death
Cannot destroy what has been given.

I am learning to look at your life again
Instead of your death and your departing.*

Special factors

The early stages of bereavement start with knowing that one (or one's partner, relation or friend) is HIV antibody positive. Some of the factors that differentiate grief over this as opposed to other diseases are:

- *Concurrent diagnosis* of being HIV positive, of developing AIDS Related Complex and the AIDS syndrome itself.
- *Suicide* is certainly considered by a great majority who are informed of the different diagnoses.
- *Co-factors.* Certainly alcohol and substance abuse as coping mechanisms may be used by the sufferer. Alcohol and substance abuse feed on the suicidal temptations.
- *Age and stage differences.* There is no doubt that most young men (and women) are not ready or equipped psychologically or developmentally to face premature death.
- *Multiple loss.* There are many today who, before having to cope with their own loss of self, are coping with the loss of a partner as well as many, many friends, and these are likely to increase. I met one man recently who had lost twelve close friends within the space of two years. The grief load for him is almost unbearable, all the more so because he too is antibody positive.
- *Legal complexities.* It often happens that, when the loved one has died, his biological family will claim all his estate, leaving his partner bereft of everything. This happens because so many partners have not made a will. Grieving partners are legally not protected if there is no will. It is essential for a will to be drawn up with the help of a solicitor, with the partner and one other being the executors. This allows for the wishes of the dying person to be fulfilled and enables the surviving partner to make all funeral arrangements and to attend.

* Marjorie Pizer, *To You the Living* (Second Back Row Press, NSW, Australia, 1981).

- *Acute fear and anxiety* is natural when one realises that many of these PLW/HIV are anticipating their own impending diagnosis and death, complicated by the fact that they may have infected another. Partners are potentially at risk of positive diagnosis within the HIV infection, ARC, AIDS continuum.
- *Differentiation* between somatic symptoms of normal anxiety and symptoms of the possible disease. Every spot, mark, pain is analysed minutely as a possible sign of growing infection.
- *Lack of biological family support* as well as traditional institutional and community support. The traditional rituals around grief and loss are often inappropriate to meet the needs of HIV infected persons, most of whom in the West, at present, are members of the gay community.
- *Lack of spiritual support.* This is partly due to the fact that many members of the gay community have been in the past, and still are in many instances, ostracised by the Church as a whole. As a result they are unlikely to turn to the Church for comfort, with the added danger of further rejection. There is no doubt many do turn to other faiths or sects for the spiritual support of acceptance.
- *Community services* are developing mainly from within the gay community itself, the forerunner in care and educational programmes. Among the services offered by the Terrence Higgins Trust are the 'Buddy System' (support for sufferers on a one-to-one basis) and specialist support groups such as 'Body Positive' and 'Frontliners' who offer care in the community to those infected with the virus and who are themselves actually living with ARC or AIDS. Increasingly, local authorities are incorporating the needs of PLW/HIV into their social services by offering home-helps and meals-on-wheels. In fact, voluntary and statutory organisations in different areas are coming together to co-ordinate a network of varying care services. This will become a reality when both types of organisation recognise and accept their need for each other in providing care for all involved in the different stages of this infection.
- *Secrecy* and isolation are used as coping mechanisms by the family to protect itself from rejection and ostracism from

within itself, from neighbours and from the workplace. One minister, on being informed by a mother that her son was at home dying of AIDS, refused to bring him communion or to allow him to be buried from his church. Employers have found ways of releasing PLW/HIV from their employ, including those who associate with them. Increasingly insurance companies are devising questionnaires in order to find out who are and who are not at risk of infection.

Counselling bereaved partners, relatives and friends

When two people who love each other are separated by the death of one, the survivor normally becomes host to a number of confusing thoughts and feelings that ebb and flow without any apparent predictability. Certainly there is grief, one of life's most profound emotional experiences, but grief can also be a celebration that the dying is over, even if there are periods of loneliness, memories and heartache yet to come. The grieving period (or its immediate aftermath) is a time of transition, within which one reassesses one's own beliefs, philosophies, relationships to others and to the rest of the world. During this very sensitive and vulnerable period, the survivor can expect to feel tearful, misunderstood (by those who have not suffered loss), guilty (for no good reason) and angry with those who fail to understand that the loss of a gay partner can be just as devastating as the loss of a non-gay partner.

A great majority of survivors of partners who have died from this viral infection are young people who have not experienced mortal loss previously. This makes their pain all the more confusing for them. Many of the deceased are youths and their dying seems to have served no purpose. It is not uncommon to hear the bereaved say 'I'm going mad'. All the minister or other carer can do is offer his or her presence to the person who is suffering the loss of a loved one to AIDS.

Denial is one of the grief characteristics experienced by male partners of men in the gay community, which is itself being forced to become more and more expert in handling the different stages of bereavement. The bereaved man will complain that his friends are getting tired of hearing him talk about his partner and that they are pressurising him to let his partner go. 'How can you continue to imprison your partner's soul by wishing he was still beside you?'

When beginning to care for the bereaved man, it is necessary to encourage him to use whatever time he needs to talk about, to think about, have erotic fantasies about, or cry about, the loss of his partner. We must make time to be 'with' the person or not be there at all. It is essential to give him permission to talk about AIDS, whatever the gay man's friends may have said, and not to allow him to hurry the process of a bereavement which they may well find hard to handle.

After the funeral or cremation, the partner may become more immediately aware of his own susceptibility to AIDS. This is a contagion of fear that he can suspend for a time in order to remain close to his dying friend, but afterwards he is likely to find it coming back rather strongly. The bereaved partner is now aware of what AIDS looks like and may be terrified of getting it from, or giving it to, anyone else. Consequently, sexual repression and anxiety about contagion and infection are strong.

AIDS is mysterious and therefore frightening. Society as a whole is afraid of it and does not want to be reminded of or be touched by it. The bereaved partner, therefore, may often feel stigmatised by his association with his partner. On becoming aware that he is HIV or seropositive, there arises the question and the guilt as to whether or not he infected his partner. The simple offering of the embrace of understanding and compassion can be of immense help here to soften the feelings of leprous alienation of self by self or by others. Since the disease kept the partner on an exhausting schedule before the death, and since he was too busy to worry about dating and safer sex, he will now need reassurance that he is capable of being close to men physically without exposure to, or transmission of, the HIV virus.

Many who were primarily responsible for the day-to-day care of their partners have a much more difficult time emotionally after the funeral, particularly if they had conflicts with the partner's family about his care. Gay partners often have to fight the family for acceptance of the primacy of their bond and the independence of their relationship.

All partners tend to be idealistic, particularly in the early stages of the relationship. In these circumstances, a rigid idealisation of the dead partner can occur, causing new male friends to be unwelcomed: 'Nobody can be as good as my lover.' While saying this, and in a way denying the need for a relationship, the bereaved longs for the closeness and the support he gave to his dying partner. In the last stages of his life, the person with AIDS and his partner will often return to the romantic stage when they were greatly in love with each other.

The problem then is that, when the partner dies, he leaves behind a devoted 'widower', if one can use that term within the context of a gay bereavement.

We need to remember in our caring that many gay partners have experienced the full ingredients of a loving monogamous relationship – devotion, putting the other person first, seeing the best of oneself in the other person. As most of these relationships grow in depth, a working balance of autonomy and independence is negotiated, and we are witness to the fact that it is not only a relationship of mutual interdependence but also rich in its co-creative potential. However, it is because of the great dependency of those dying from AIDS/ARC, the youthfulness of the men it attacks, and the untimely interruption to the intimacy that a partner's death brings, that he who is left behind will need to be helped to regain his autonomy. Although he has a need for companionship, he in some way awaits his departed partner's approval.

It does appear that those who are involved with HIV care activities recover more quickly from the death of their partners. This is perhaps because many of the volunteers they may be working with will have been through similar experiences and therefore 'know' in a way that the minister cannot unless he himself is infected.

Recently I had the privilege (as it always is) to celebrate at a cremation service. This service echoed all the love that the man had received up to the moment of his dying, tended as he was by his family and friends. His parents, originally unaware of their son's sexual orientation, were shattered when this was discovered. Fortunately this pain of discovery was eased by the fact that their son was constantly cared for day and night by his friends. The parents were overwhelmed by the love their son received. 'We have never seen nor experienced such loving.' The singing of 'All things bright and beautiful' (as requested by their son) lifted the veil of bereavement and exposed the mystery of hope 'that all shall be well and all shall be well and all manner of things shall be well.'*

Helping the family to understand and cope

There is no one answer, no one particular piece of advice that I know of, that will enable the family, especially the male members, to cope with the full ramifications of AIDS. It is important for me to remember how difficult it must be to grasp the fact that, for the first time, family members (especially parents) are being informed not only that their son is gay, but that he has a lover and that he is probably dying of a disease which they will consider need never have happened.

Often the immediate response is one of shock, of anger and disgust. The father and other close male members of the family may well feel their own maleness is being questioned. Questions arise in the mind: 'Where did we go wrong?' 'What have I produced?' 'As he is my son or brother, does that mean I could be gay also?' 'What will the neighbours think?' These questions are often compounded by a sense of guilt, helplessness and inadequacy. There is a tendency to blame the partner for infecting the son, because parents cannot accept the fact that their son may have had several partners over the years. The knowledge that they did not really know their son and that he feared informing them of his lifestyle poses the question: 'Why could he not trust us?'

Initially what is needed, in my experience, is the space of time for the family, especially the male members, to be able to express their pain at what is happening to themselves as well as to their son. Space to be angry, to voice confusion, is essential, and is far more beneficial than any so-called 'right

* Julian of Norwich, *Revelations of Divine Love.*

answers'. We are there at the edge of their pain to be a recipient of their shock, whatever its form or nature. We embrace them as we would any other person who feels they are losing a part of themselves or fears that they themselves will be infected with this viral infection.

While the male members of the family for the most part have great difficulty in coping with their son's or brother's gayness, his partner and his dying, the female members (i.e. the mother or sister), after the initial shock, appear better able to accept the situation and often help in looking after the son or brother and his partner.

It is possible to help the whole family through their pain by encouraging them to share with their son's partner and friends in caring for him, whether at his and his partner's home, or at the hospital or hospice. In so doing their stereotyped image of gay men is changed, as they witness the loving care of those who are sharing in their son's needs. These same men are very often found caring for the parents, too, as they have some awareness of what their friend's family may be going through.

The only way I have been able to be of any real assistance in these circumstances is by being the bridging person between the son, his partner and their respective parents, being available to them in their different needs. So often my quiet presence is all that can be coped with, as I wait for the invitation to move in closer, literally to embrace and be embraced by the parents. I move in closer, as it were, with the truths of the situation for all concerned. Therefore, as a person of authority in their eyes, I can help them to be aware of the fact that their son's gayness is neither a fault of theirs nor of his. His sexual orientation was probably well established before puberty. Equally, their feelings of anger and rage are of no help to their son, and if they accept all of their son – his total being – they will see that they have every reason to be proud of him and to love him, so that he may die knowing that he is accepted and loved by them unconditionally.

One of the more unpleasant jokes about AIDS describes the gay man confronting his parents with good news and bad news; first the bad news that the son is gay; then the good news that he is dying of AIDS. Such jokes clearly reflect the stigmatising nature of society's attitude towards homosexuality and, by association, HIV infection. They make fun of the triple adjustment that families have to undergo in coping with a son who has AIDS. Unfortunately, these three facts are forced into parents' awareness at the same time: your son is gay, your son has a partner and your son is dying. This knowledge can, and often does, create an immense amount of conflict and trauma for the parents and for other members of the family. In families where the son's sexual identity was unknown before the onset of terminal AIDS the level of denial is probably at first quite high. In such situations, it is the work of the minister and other carers to help parents confront the psychological pain associated with this news. Where these basic conflicts are resolved, parents may then begin to approach their son with more love and support and stay close through his illness, an illness which may change the very fabric of their relationship with him as well as changing the fabric of relationships throughout the whole family.

In many cases it is the mother who can cope best. One man spent two hours with his mother after he had told her that he had Kaposi's sarcoma. He wanted all the members of his family to know. His mother took the opposite view, fearing stigmatisation of herself and her family. He, however, insisted that they should be told. It was important to his physical and mental health that he should be supported by all who truthfully loved him. For him it was a test of whose love was unconditional. Finally, his mother relented. He then discovered, after telling the other members of his family of his sexual orientation and diagnosis, that they all appeared to know of his homosexuality but had been concerned for his parents and agreed to a conspiracy of silence. Certainly it helps all concerned if families are aware of these facts and then, if the man has a partner, they can appreciate his place in their son's life. It is well known that any painful event is best dealt with if held in the light of truth and not hidden away in the darkness of fear. Grief has a secretive and depressing, special and private, flavour which usually dissipates when someone else is allowed into the grieving processes.

One mother resolved her denial of her son's homosexual orientation by throwing a large birthday party for him in his community and inviting his friends. She moved closer to her son because of the love with which he was surrounded. As a result, the love his friends had for her son expressed itself by including her in recognition of the overtures she had been prepared to make.

Many young men, after leaving the family home for whatever reasons, develop a new 'chosen family' of significant people and will usually rally round to assist the person who is ill with social, financial and supportive help of various kinds. In a smooth process after death, this network of friends and, one hopes, the dead man's natural family can share their ritual of grieving together. One mother and father, coming away from their son's memorial service, could only say, 'We always knew our son was loved and lovable'.

Unfortunately, some families are unable to cross the boundaries of fear and misunderstanding. This occurs when they create ritual and personal grief processes that exclude friends of the gay man. While this may be a natural reaction when the family is in a state of shock, it is also painfully alienating. It has been known for the partner to be banned from the crematorium or funeral which had been closed to everyone but the 'immediate family'. Two men may live together for twenty years and share everything but, in death, the survivor finds that he has no sanctions, social or legal. He may also be denied bereavement leave by his employer. If the family does not recognise the validity of their gay son's life style, or the rights of his chosen partner to grieve (preferably with them), or to share in making decisions regarding the estate, then conflict can result. The situation can then become extremely volatile, given the stress felt by all concerned. When such situations occur the minister or other carer may find themselves acting as a mediator, attempting both to smooth the necessary transitional stages and also to cushion the anger and guilt by promoting an understanding of the basis of these feelings which may be a manifestation of much which lies below the surface.

Like war, this viral infection is taking young persons from their families, their partners. 'It's not supposed to happen this way' and 'He is supposed to bury me, not me him' are statements I hear. Facing a death in the family, especially if the person is dying of AIDS and is young, is perhaps the most difficult of deaths to face. Mercifully, accepting the truth into oneself and offering it to others contribute to easing this almost unbearable pain. The following article, entitled 'Merciful Truths', helps us to recognise how one couple found that their honesty brought comfort.

The Schows' letter begins: 'Dear Friends, we are writing this to let you know that Brad, our eldest son, passed away on Friday, December 5. Prior to his death, he asked that there be no public announcement of the fact and that there be no funeral; we intend to honour these requests. But since you are among those who care for him and for us, we want you to know something of the circumstances of a life which ended prematurely.

'There were several physical conditions that contributed to Brad's demise, all of which are traceable to an undermined immune system. He had AIDS, a fact of which he and we became aware in the summer of 1985.'

The parents describe how in June 1985 Brad came home from his studies at Utah State University to help them build a new house. When he became too ill to help, he stayed with his parents for the next year and a half. Following an appendectomy that summer, his condition worsened. Pneumocystis pneumonia crept up on him and the AIDS diagnosis was confirmed.

'You could not call him lucky, but he was, at least, more fortunate than some AIDS victims. He did not develop Kaposi's sarcoma, the skin cancer that often occurs with AIDS. Although he lost the sight in one eye towards the end, and experienced limited paralysis and, of course, dramatic loss of strength and weight, his mind remained alert and clear virtually to the end.

'That extra year, granted after [his] near-death in November 1985, was a gift to him as well as to us. We will not forget the conversations he had as the days and nights passed . . . It was a time of profound emotional and spiritual significance for all of us.'

After it became impossible for the Schows to provide for their son's medical needs at home, he went back to hospital. 'The end was not easy, but there were some periods of tranquillity for him during the last several days. We were with him when he died. He had wished to be cremated, so we helped to prepare him in the clothing he had chosen. At this point we stood as a family round his hospital bed and thanked God for the gift of Brad's life among us.'

This letter seems to me a good example, even for unbelievers, of the truth being merciful. After reading it one feels sorry for parents who have had to concoct elaborate lies about the deaths of their children of AIDS, or who have reacted to the general hysteria about the disease itself by not allowing their children to come home.

The Schows ended their letter by saying: 'We are proud of our son and of the courage and integrity with which he faced the difficult circumstances of his life. In this, we refer not only to his terminal illness but also the fact of his homosexuality of which we have known for eight years. Our experience during that time has taught us that society generally and organised religions in particular have much to answer for in their treatment of homosexual men and women.'

Americans tend to be more open about their deepest emotions, says David Miller, an AIDS counsellor and clinical psychologist at the Middlesex Hospital Medical School, who finds it hard to imagine an English family writing such a letter. In England, he says, although it seems that few families have rejected relatives with AIDS, and most have been privately supportive, very few go public because they fear that friends and colleagues will reject them if they do tell the truth.

Wayne Schow, a professor of English at Idaho State University, said writing the letter had proved a cathartic experience for him and his wife: 'We asked Brad before he died how we could show our feelings about him. He said, "If you want, have a wake for me." But it was a bad social mix for a party: Mormon officials, gay friends from LA, local people, some of whom are very conservative. Besides,

57

we had been through an ordeal and we didn't feel like hosting anything.

'But we did want the world to know we were proud of him and his life, and we didn't want it swept under the carpet. When the letters came back, we realised how wonderful it is simply to be supported by people when you have been through an ordeal; so many people were fond of Brad.'*

This true story gives us hope while at the same time removing the stigma of AIDS; to die of an opportunistic infection due to immune deficiency is no worse and no better than dying of some other illness. It is important to remember that *no one* dies of ARC/AIDS itself.

Caring for the dying

It is because dying is the inevitable outcome of this infection that it seems right to offer some guidelines to help us understand and care for the loved one who is dying. Who better to guide us than Elisabeth Kübler-Ross who with others has added her own insight to the pioneer work of caring for the dying. We expect such care for the new born. Why should we not expect it for the dying, who are being born, perhaps, into the greater life, the greater mystery, of death into life?

Elisabeth Kübler-Ross† reminds us of the five different attitudes of the dying person, to which I dare to add a sixth – *Waiting*. These attitudes may occur at any time within a matter of hours. Different carers may elicit different responses.

1 *Denial*: 'No, not me.' This is a typical reaction when a person learns that he or she is terminally ill. Denial is important and necessary. It helps cushion the impact of the patient's awareness that death is inevitable.

2 *Rage and anger*: 'Why me?' The person resents the fact that others will remain healthy and alive while he or she must die. God is a special target for anger, since he is regarded as imposing, arbitrarily, the death sentence. To those who are

* Julia Orange, *The Times*, 2 March 1987.
† Elisabeth Kübler-Ross, *On Death and Dying* (Tavistock, 1970).

shocked at her claim that such anger is not only permissible but inevitable, Dr Kübler-Ross replies succinctly, 'God can take it.'

3 *Bargaining*: 'Yes me, but . . .' The person accepts the fact of death but strikes bargains for more time. Mostly they bargain with God – even people who never talked about or with God before. They promise to be good or to do something in exchange for another week or month or year of life. Notes Dr Kübler-Ross: 'What they promise is totally irrelevant, because they don't keep their promises anyway.'

4 *Depression*: 'Yes, me.' First, the person mourns past losses, things not done, wrongs committed. But then he or she enters a state of 'preparatory grief', getting ready for the arrival of death. The patient grows quiet, doesn't want visitors. 'When a dying patient doesn't want to see you any more', says Dr Kübler-Ross 'this is a sign he has finished his unfinished business with you, and it is a blessing. He can now let go peacefully.'

5 *Acceptance*: 'My time is very close now and it's all right.' Dr Kübler-Ross describes this final stage as 'not a happy stage, but neither is it unhappy. It's devoid of feelings but it's not resignation; it's really a victory.' As one person recently said to me, 'It's okay. I have made peace with God, with myself and my friends. I can hardly wait. I'm so excited.'

6 *Waiting*: This, I believe, is the stage before the actual dying. This statement was from a person to whom I was offering pastoral care. 'I'm *waiting* for the plane to take off into the mystery.'

These stages provide a very useful guide to understanding the different phases dying people may go through. They are not absolute; not everyone goes through every stage, in this exact sequence, at some predictable pace. But this paradigm can, if used in a flexible, insight-producing way, be a valuable tool in understanding why a patient may be behaving as he or she does.

Dying is a mystery. We are angry because we often feel so helpless when faced by its reality as we grow with dying people in our understanding of death. The light of Christ's death and resurrection acknowledges the fact that, in them, as in all of us, are the seeds of the crucifixion and the resurrection: the final stages of growth are a dying into a completeness of life.

Those suffering from HIV infection are facing two deaths:

1 The death of 'coming out' and facing their homosexuality or bisexuality with all the shame, guilt and rejection with which society has invested them.

2 Their impending death and how that may take place, enhanced by fears of aloneness, pain, rejection, disfigurement, loss of control both mentally and physically, and a pervading sense of uselessness.

Many who are living with HIV infection will, during the course of their illness, seek pastoral and spiritual support either from other faiths, often Zen Buddhism, or faith healers before seeking help from the Church because many have been ostracised by the institution that *still condemns them*. It is felt that pastoral care is given, not with love, but rather because 'the minister has to; it is his duty'. Yet many who are ill seek out the Christian minister who will quietly visit, embrace and pray with them as they prepare for a healing, even if it be a healing unto death.

Many making this journey into healing unto death need constant assurance about the following:

- that they will be as free as possible of pain
- that they will die with dignity
- that they will die surrounded by the most significant people in their life
- that they will find some answer to the question: 'What happens to me when I die?'

For all, whether Christian or not, there is the question, 'Am I acceptable to God?' It is important for all to have an awareness that none is excluded from the love of God. What is needed is the affirming act of authentication to themselves that they are of value even in their dying.

Sufferers in the terminal (or near terminal) stages of dying should have a say in where they would like this to take place, usually in their own home, fully supported by their partner and family, where possible.

We must also help them to realise that

it is never too late to put things right in their relationships. Like ourselves, most sufferers do not want to die, nor want the people closest to them to die, without first re-establishing the deepest possible connection with each other. The sooner we take whatever initiative is necessary to accomplish this, the less costly the separation will be for all concerned. We should live every day in such a way that, if the people who have been closest to us were to die, we would have no reason to reproach ourselves for things we did not say or do.*

It is important that we enable the partner (or other significant people) to be involved with the person's dying as together they prepare for a co-creative letting go of each other. This means, I suggest, that we recognise the unrecognised rights of the partner, similar to the common law situation in Scotland. The partner will want all the support possible, for many have no family support, unless they happen to be linked into a group of friends who, over the years, have become their 'natural family' through friendships shared.

If the minister has been able to 'walk with' the person who has died, he or she will have come to know who has meant most to that person in his or her life. During the time of preparing for death, the deceased will have been encouraged to sort out his or her life with the partner and with others who are close.

Whatever the attitude of the Church minister, the transmission of the *love* of God is in the *embrace of the touch*, in the *activity of prayer* and in the *silent offering* of the words of love that *do not require prior penitence*. It requires only the presence of another vulnerable human person who has the courage of faith to allow for the mutuality of care between them to take place. The minister must be prepared simply to sit and to *be* alongside the partner and the person who is dying. The 'touch of presence' will increase the sense of being acceptable as he or she flows into the mystery of death: the completeness of life.

* From a Funeral Service Programme. Author anonymous.

To die of cancer is to die surrounded, in most instances, with the compassion of love's enfoldingness. However, to die through being infected with the HIV virus, transmitted as it is through bodily fluids, especially semen and blood, is to die, in many instances, involved in one's own fears of being unwanted, of being a nobody, of being a leper. This is often confirmed by the fears and by the anger of others, especially those who should be close.

To die feeling like a leper is a psychological wound that is almost beyond repair and is nearly always caused by unthinking attitudes and uncaring behaviour. We need to assist the partner and the one who is dying to recognise not only each other's painful needs but also those of their respective families. As I have illustrated earlier, the dying man can be surrounded by one of two extremes:

1 A father refusing to accept his son and doing all he can to prevent his son's partner from attending the funeral. This of course creates a situation of hatred that can be mutual, as neither is able to recognise the other's pain. It is pain hammering against pain.

2 The young man dying with his partner holding one hand, his mother holding the other and his father embracing them all. They have mutually recognised the dignity of the relationship, hence a mutual sharing of the pain – love reaching in love to love.

Only the compassion of love's empathy will enable us to embrace both the above situations and to know that all shall be well, for in the ending is to be found a new beginning.

Lord, now lettest thou thy servant depart in peace. (Luke 2:29)

In the ending is my beginning. (T. S. Eliot)

7

Rites of Passage

Worship cares for us

The term 'rite of passage' was first coined by the French anthropologist Arnold van Gennep in 1909 because he became increasingly aware that the life of every individual consists of 'a series of passages from one age to another and from one occupation to another'. A person's life 'comes to be made up of a succession of stages with similar ends and beginnings: birth, puberty, marriage, fatherhood (motherhood) and special relationship bondings (formal and informal), occupational specialisation (and retirement), and death'. He goes on to say: 'For every one of these events, there are ceremonies whose essential purpose is to enable the individual to pass from one defined position to another which is equally well defined.'*

As ministers, we know there is a need for rituals, and none are more essential than those for grief. Van Gennep has classified these into three successive stages: separation, transition and re-entering. 'These rites of passage facilitate a person's transition from one life stage to another.' We need to be aware that grieving is *not* simply about the present, it is also about the loss of the past and the future. When someone has died through AIDS, rites communicate to the individual's community the new status or role of the survivng partner of a gay or lesbian relationship, a role which may not always be recognised by families or others associated with the grieving gay man or woman. These rites provide for emotional

---

* Arnold van Gennep, *On Rites of Passage* (University of Chicago Press, 1980).

release, offering the partner the same opportunity to deal directly with his or her loss and with the emotions involved. They provide an acceptable framework within which to grieve. Sadly this is seldom possible for the gay partner who is so often isolated from involvement in the funeral arrangements and the funeral itself, and who may not be invited to the funeral breakfast.

Rituals, at their best, link our individual experiences with not only the corporate experience of the community, but also the universal experiences of all humankind. When they are offered with the majesty of simplicity they encourage people to confront the reality of their loss and their emotions surrounding that loss in a co-healing manner. This enables those who are grieving to come together again enriched by the experience and to be authenticated in an ongoing co-creative manner. However it is essential that these liturgies are chosen with care and are not empty ceremonies. As Robin Green states:

> Worship cares for us. Inappropriate liturgy can strip us of our sense of worth and dignity. The case study raises some basic issues about the relationship of worship and pastoral care. Those issues include the importance of continuity and familiarity; the appropriateness of different liturgies for different groups; the relationship of image and symbol to human needs; the ways in which the proclamation of the Word of God connects with actual human experience.*

R. Scott Sullender goes further:

> As we work with grieving people, we must be keenly aware of the sense of drama in their lives. We must not see them just as a case or as a generalised type, but as unique individuals with their own encounters with God, temptations, defeats, and victories. We must place whatever present loss we are dealing with in the context of the whole sweep of the person's life. We must grasp the whole, the flow of their lives, the process of their struggling towards salvation.†

* Robin Green, *Only Connect* (Darton, Longman & Todd, 1987).
† R. Scott Sullender, *Grief and Growth* (Paulist Press, 1985).

The spoken word of the homily at the funeral service is crucial. It is therefore essential for the minister to meet the most relevant person in the deceased's life, ideally before his death, and to hear from others who mattered, including the dying man himself, about his journeying in and through life to his dying into life. In this way, we authenticate his presence in the world now and his presence in the mystery labelled 'death'.

Only in this way can we enable the bereaved to remove blockages to the co-creative grieving that should flow into their lives. This task is theirs to fulfil: to meet and to strive for the growth potential which is seeded in the grieving heart. It is through ritual that we are linked to the uniqueness of each person's drama and, with them, find ourselves incorporated into the larger dramas of all humankind, whatever their faith or non-faith. If we have loved hard, we should expect to grieve hard.

The minister's acquaintance with grief will enable him or her to offer the gift of co-creative empathy, in the realisation that one person's sorrow is also another's. A rite should be a celebration of *love*.

It is the comfort of the liturgies of silence and touch, of just being present, which is helpful to the dying person and those releasing him into the greater dimensions of moving into 'My Father's house' where 'there are many mansions'. These liturgies may begin during the pre-bereavement times through services, such as the laying-on of hands, anointing, the ritual of reconciliation.

All services should be conducted with the dignity we would offer anyone whatever their illness. We must not be pressurised into getting it over with as soon as possible. 'Hurry up – you know what's in there.' It is crucial that we remind ourselves that the healing of grief begins at the latest at the funeral, cremation or memorial service. We must not let the fears, the anxieties, the possible shame or guilt which may be around prevent the rituals of bereavement and death being sensitively prepared and offered.

Often a memorial service is requested by the family or friends. Sometimes it is requested by those who were unable to be at the funeral, either because it took place in another part of the country or because the son's or daughter's parents refused to allow the gay men and women friends to attend, not wanting the family or their friends to know of their son's or daughter's gayness and to prevent suspicion that the son or daughter has died of AIDS.

The rituals, the rites of worship, are essential to life. One might even say that without the rituals in life to life we are as dead. They centre our lives and bring a fullness to them. Rituals go deep and one cannot play around with their sacredness. As James Roose-Evans says:

> A ritual puts one in touch with the elemental and the transcendental, with that which is deep within us and that which is beyond us and which we call God . . . Certain rituals are timeless, shaped, perfected and handed across the centuries (and the differing faiths) in the form of great liturgies. Other rituals are co-created for a specific need, time and space.*

And as Peter Shaffer said in *Equus*: 'If you do not worship you'll shrink, it's as brutal as that.'

---

* James Roose-Evans, *Inner Journey, Outer Journey* (Rider, 1987).

8

Living our Dyings

Awareness of one's own dying

As ministers, we must be aware of the potential of our own mortality and be prepared to examine how we have coped with the many dying experiences in our own daily progress towards death. This self-examination will make us all the more able to assist the sick person in his or her pilgrimage into the greater mystery. Most of us have died many times during our lives. Every major change is a form of dying, also the various disappointments in our life. We are born to die that we might live into the mystery of all life, visible and invisible.

It is important that I should again stress the following points:

- We need to be aware of, and to be psychologically comfortable with, the dying and with those who are in the process of becoming bereaved.
- We can only risk being emotionally acceptable to the person of our concern if we are able to confront fears about our own dying. I ask myself, have I the courage of faith to recognise myself in the sufferer, who is also in me? When this occurs, the barriers of professionalism vanish.
- To deny any emotional connection with the dying person is to increase the violence of his or her disease.

To help us come to terms with our own daily and terminal dying, which began at the moment of our birth into this dimension of our being, the following questions might concentrate our minds co-creatively. Questions similar to these were given to me on a retreat, but unfortunately I do not know

67

the source. My answers were quite enlightening to me if to no one else!

- Whom would you like to be at your side when you are dying?
- Who will miss you?
- What impression would you like to leave behind when you die?
- What have you to put right with yourself before you die?
- What relationships have you to put right before you die?
- Whom have you to say 'thanks' to for whatever?
- Who should know how much you love them?
- From whom should you seek forgiveness and with whom reconciliation?
- To whom should you offer forgiveness?
- What do you want to achieve before you die?
- What kind of funeral or memorial service would you like and whom would you specially invite?

Anthony de Mello* suggests exercises to help us deal with our own dying, so that we may be all the more able to help one another, so long as we accept the fact that each person's death belongs to that person, who must be allowed to journey into it in his or her own way and space of timing. The exercises he suggests are:

- seeing life in perspective
- saying goodbye to your body
- being at your funeral
- fantasy on the corpse
- consciousness of the past

It is perhaps even more crucial in this particular kind of ministry that we understand ourselves. We must learn to know and to acknowledge our own feelings about dying and the many forms and causes of death. These feelings will affect our work. Their effect can be positive if we are truthful about them and know how to ventilate them co-creatively. Let us not forget that the energy expended in hiding and suppressing our feelings is energy taken away from using and offering our

* Anthony de Mello, *Sadhana - a way to God* (Doubleday, 1984 edn).

knowledge and skills co-creatively. To the extent that we can deal with our own fears and anxieties about our own dying and mortality, so we shall enable the dying person to do likewise. Death is the ultimate liberator, releasing us into a wholeness of being, of completeness.

Being with the dying and the bereaved, whatever the nature of the illness and whoever the bereaved are, includes living with the dying and the bereaved for different lengths of time. This means living with the truth that I must die also, and that I *am* dying as I continue the journey that is unending, as I flow with others into the unknown.

The harvest of death is life

'Faith, hope and love' are the substance of life unto death and death unto life – especially love. Recently I received a small card with these words by Edith Sitwell: 'Love is not changed by death and nothing is lost and all in the end is harvest.' This is why it is crucial for those of us who are given the privilege to be with the dying and the bereaved to assist such persons to realise that nothing is wasted and that all is caught up in the ongoing creativeness of God and the ongoing co-creative potential of every man, woman and child. Death and life are two sides of the same coin. Death belongs to life as birth does in initiating us into this life.

Our basic ministry with the dying and the bereaved *is to listen*, to listen *attentively*, with such care that the dying and the bereaved can listen comfortably to themselves and flow into the future with confidence, the confidence that comes through being authenticated, of having given the world something that is specifically theirs, not ours.

Life is for dying, and dying is for living and loving of the kind that will enable all concerned to 'fear forward' out of the darkness of their pain into the brightness of a healing that will, once again, release the mystery of their co-creative potential.

We should encourage everyone to live in the knowledge that our loved ones

　　have only slipped away into the next room. I am I and you

69

are you. Whatever we were to each other that we are still. Call me by my old familiar name, speak to me in the easy way which you always used. Put no difference into your tone; wear no forced air of solemnity or sorrow. Laugh as we always laughed at the little jokes we enjoyed together. Play, smile, think of me, pray for me. Let my name be ever the household word that it always was. Let it be spoken without effort, without the ghost of a shadow on it. Life means all that it ever meant. It is the same as it ever was; there is absolutely unbroken continuity. Why should I be out of mind because I am out of sight? I am waiting for you, for an interval, somewhere very near just around the corner. All is well.*

I suggest that the problem of death is not usually the person dying, but rather those who are in the process of becoming bereaved. In my experience, the majority of those who have allowed me to be a witness and an enabler in their movement towards dying are not worried about death itself. Most are saddened by what they feel is the incompleteness of their lives on many levels, especially that of self-fulfilment. This is because many of the dying have been dominated by other people's versions of how they should have fulfilled their lives. So often, the young person has not lived long enough to move out of parental and other parental-type authority. It takes a very strong person to fulfil his or her life through activities that are self-authenticating rather than other-authenticating.

It is one of the functions of the ministry to encourage this self-authenticating process in the dying person, as he or she authenticates the co-creative potential of death through being fully aware of his or her dying and actively taking part in the whole process of treatment and care. This will be possible only if we cease to put time limits on each person's life. As ministers, we are expected to help ourselves and all those with whom we come in contact to realise that it is the 'quality' rather than the 'quantity' of life that is so important. I have found that persons infected with HIV will speak of the quality rather than the length of their lives. For many it is the depth

* Written by Canon Henry Scott Holland (1847–1918)

of friendship shared that really matters, not the number of acquaintances.

It is my experience that when a person is strong enough to have accepted life in all its joys and pains (and this includes accepting that his or her dying to that life is the very reason for living), then the dying process is being authenticated. An even stronger encouragement to make something of one's life can remove all fear of death, though it may not remove the pains of sadness, of departing from all those who have become a part of the fabric of one's life.

When this occurs at whatever age; and it does occur with some young people – there has been a triumph over death. One could say, in fact, life continues to triumph over death. We can help the person to recognise that he or she has completed the life seeded within at birth, a life now being released into the mystery of a future that is beyond our comprehension, into the greatest 'cloud of unknowing'.

Unless ministers can sense and *be* the meaning of their own lives, they will not enter into the meaning of another's life no matter what its shortness or length. All have the potential for living a lifetime in the moment of *now*, whether that *now* be of a day's duration, of a year's duration or of many years' duration.

What does matter is how richly one lives the time of *now*. We need to remember that time is relative, that the length of our years is relative. What is crucial is the positiveness of those years, of the time allotted to each person. Each person is of course different, because each, we hope, has been allowed and encouraged all through his or her own life to do his or her 'own thing' with an integrity of purpose. This is not only self-authenticating and self-fulfilling but also co-creative.

Our work as ministers is to encourage the co-creative potential of every death – of every dying into the mystery of whatever is to come – through the mystery of love's endeavouring as we enable each other to complete the incompleteness of our lives. The completeness of life is the death of life as we know it into the life of love's mystery unending.

As Elisabeth Kübler-Ross states:

Death is the final stage of growth in this life. There is no total

71

death. Only the body dies. The self or spirit, or whatever you may wish to label it, is eternal. You may interpret this in any way that makes you comfortable.

If you wish, you may view the eternal essence of your existence in terms of the impact your every mood and action has on those you touch, and then in turn, on those they touch, and on and on – even after your life span is completed. You will never know, for example, the rippling effects of the smile and words of encouragement you give to other human beings with whom you come in contact.

You may be more comfortable and comforted by a faith that is a source of goodness, light and strength greater than any of us individually, yet still within us all, and that each essential self has an existence that transcends the finiteness of the physical and contributes to that greater power.

Death, in this context, may be viewed as the curtain between the existence that we are conscious of and one that is hidden from us until we raise that curtain. Whether we open it symbolically in order to understand the finiteness of the existence we know, thus learning to live each day the best we can, or whether we open it in actuality when we end that physical existence is not the issue. What is important is to realise that whether we understand fully why we are here or what will happen when we die, it is our purpose as human beings to grow – to look within ourselves to find and build upon that source of peace and understanding and strength which is our inner selves and to reach out to others with love, acceptance, patient guidance, and hope for what we all may become together.*

The death of each person signifies that the work of love is finished for him or her in this dimension of being, for themselves, for others and for God, our ultimate lover.

---

* Elisabeth Kübler-Ross, *Death, the Final Stage of Growth* (Simon & Schuster, 1986).

9

Ministers and Other Carers

At a conference for ministers, Peter Randall, a person living
with AIDS, said: 'We don't need your theology. What we
need is your healing.' We will only be able to respond if
we are able to hear through our listening. It is crucial that
we should be able to hear what help the people we are
concerned with require, not what we, with the bias of our
own needs, think is needed. We must hear what permission
is being given us to release their potential for change, for
growth. This will come through the strengths of their weaknesses, of their pain and its meaning. The more deeply we
listen, the more we shall tune in to the other person, to the
causes of suffering and to the different ways of coming to
terms with it.

In listening with others, we are enabling each person to
know who he or she is. In so doing, we are confronted with
the problems of instant labelling, either by ourselves or by
the person of our concern. Take, for instance, the person
labelled 'AIDS victim'. Without thinking or listening, we
label this person 'homosexual' when, in fact, the AIDS
sufferer could have been infected through some other form of
sexual encounter. However, if we take the time to listen to
the person behind the label, we will often hear the story of
someone wounded by members of his or her own family, who
themselves may have been too hurt to offer their children the
co-creativeness of love.

In these circumstances anyone who offers the façade of love
is welcomed as someone who may help us to forget the pain
of being unwanted and unemployed. We are often searching
for a genuine loving relationship which will draw us away
from a potentially destructive lifestyle into one that affirms

73

the mystery of our hidden goodness potential and is worth an unconditional loving of self and, therefore, of others.

If we take time to listen to the person behind any label, we shall hear of a quest for genuine love, someone who is searching for the real truth of his or her being, someone looking for the embrace of authentication of the kind that heals all manner of wounds (visible and invisible). But we must remember that all true listening is *under-the-surface* listening. The teachers in the Temple allowed Jesus to stay because he listened with his undivided attention and with the wholeness of his forgotten self.

In listening, we need the courage of faith and the expectancy of hope. The listener is expected to be a reflector of the inner vision hidden away in the darknesses, the wounds of the other person. Such listening enables us both to enjoy the co-creative potential of joyful thanksgiving. Whatever our age or infirmity, in this activity we are being about 'our Father's/our Mother's business'.

Only the listener who hears and who is single-minded enough to live from within the depths of love, and is constantly in a dialogue with God (the ultimate listener), will be able to say, by *being with* the other person, 'I am here with you and for you alone. I am listening to and with you, with the compassion of love's endeavouring.' Only through such 'attentive listening' will the image emerge inside oneself of the hidden potential of the person whose sacred presence is united to ours and both of us to God.

Listening is being for others within the activity of prayer, which is not only the Christian way but also the inter-faith way into all life, beginning with our own. In listening, we are saying 'Yes' to life and, through listening with others, we are encouraging them to say 'Yes' to life with all the pain of its co-creative potential. It is through listening that the *all* of life will be recognised in all its sacredness, as we live out to the best of our abilities the commandments to love God and one another as ourselves, as Christ loves us, and realise our full potential for healing seeded within all God's people.

He who lived these new commandments showed us the why, the how and the cost of hearing through listening. It is only through listening that we are able to recognise the other person as being irreplaceable, and it is through the openness of our intimacy, the intimacy of attentiveness, that we are able to link heart with heart, mind with mind and soul with soul.

To hear, we must be able to listen without planning, without analysing, without theorising or judging, as we awaken to the mystery of each other. It is in our hearing through listening that we are capable of enlightening each other into the unique fulfilment that we experience through our constancy of purpose in our commitment to ourselves, to others and to God-in-Christ.

All ministers are expected to be *listening companions* – comrades who hear and, in the hearing, activate the healing growth of the other person into the Way, the Truth and the Life that is uniquely his or hers. They should do this through a loving that is rich enough in compassion to hear the meaning that enfolds another in the mystery of life that is for sharing, not only with oneself, but with others and with God.

If the minister and other carers truly listen, he or she will not turn the sufferer into a victim but into a friend as, together, they help each other to live with the infection, realising that the sufferer is *in* the infection and that the friend is embracing the sufferer with the embrace of living friendship shared unconditionally. This is possible because each recognises the other's sacredness, the other's utter uniqueness, the other's freedom *to be* and to achieve his or her fullest potential co-creatively.

If we are to be attentively sensitive in our caring, our hearing, then it is crucial that we listen with the person living with AIDS, together we search for a meaning that is viable to the sufferer and carer alike. For me, Peter Randall, co-founder of 'Body Positive', enabled me to move some way towards this. In various conversations I have had with Peter, I can remember him saying:

> One of the major problems facing people with AIDS is for them to find a meaning in their experience which has a value and a use for him or her as well as society. In searching for this, what is needed is a space where these persons are not constantly confronted with the feelings and

attitudes of despair and hopelessness as they try to work their way through the maze of feeling, as the body becomes less useful and incapable of providing a means of self-expression. They will try to come to terms with the mind and body separation that is taking place because the body is increasingly no longer fulfilling its functions.

Peter also emphasises that the problem of coping physically, which can be exhausting, is often made worse by the constant worry of how it is affecting the people around one. The situation raises huge problems for people who want to care for and help those they love, but have to watch them change or disintegrate as they gradually move into the need for total care. There is the constant challenge of finding ways to help people feel safe while at the same time allowing them enough space to work out what their continuing worth is to themselves, to their loved ones and to society as a whole. A constant question is what, if any, is the real meaning of this potentially co-creative experience for all concerned, especially for the person infected with HIV.

Again, I remember Peter bringing me up short by his seeing the parallel between the experiences of the HIV infected person and of Christ during his long and fearful night in the Garden of Gethsemane. 'There must have come a time,' he says, 'when Christ had to face his own personal holocaust. What would you have said to comfort him, knowing that degradation, despair, isolation and ultimate death were inescapable?' The challenge to us all is finding some comfort in revealing the Christ in each person living with this infection.

Peter's answer would be, and I think it must also be *our* answer, 'I cannot take away your pain or alter what is happening to you, but I can tell you that your pain will always matter to me, and that I will always hold it in my heart as part of my life.' If we have the courage of faith to make such a commitment, then we are faced with the question of how to put it into practice, whether or not we can find a meaning for those inside their personal holocaust. Perhaps all we can say through the silences of shared hearing is that, in coming to know you and your experiences, *my life is being changed and not only my life but, equally important, my understanding.*

As a minister attempting to care sensitively for people who are infected with HIV, and as one who attempts to travel alongside them as the disease progressively develops into AIDS, *I can say that my life will never be the same.* These persons show me that, out of a despairing situation, we can find some meaning. We are being taught about the co-creativeness of different kinds of relationship of compassion, rich in the hope of love's unendingness.

Pastoral caring of the person infected with the HIV virus, ARC or AIDS demands that we care equally with, and for, the partner, their respective friends and families. All are in need of help and assistance to come to terms with the facts of this new viral disease and of its possible outcome for all concerned.

We need to assist the partners to recognise the *mutuality* both of the suffering and of the mourning process which each is going through in his or her own unique manner.

We need to assist each partner to recognise the *fear*, the anger, the guilt and the depression that they may be experiencing and to help, in so far as we are able, all concerned to be released from those emotional chains through the gift of understanding.

We need to be acutely aware of the *anxiety* and *fear* that the partner or spouse has of becoming infected himself or herself or, indeed, of having been the infector.

We need to encourage the partner or the spouse to share in the *truth* of the situation, thereby enabling them to be totally free and openly loving of each other, with the loving that embraces all pain, while casting out all fears.

We need to be aware of the many gay men and women who do not have a special friend, partner or spouse. It is also important to be aware of others who are *outside* the gay community (like the intravenous drug user, the haemophiliac, the pregnant lady, the small infant), who may have been infected with the HIV virus.

In caring with, and for, the family, I must emphasise again that it is important to be acutely aware that they may well be having to come to terms with their son's or daughter's homosexual or bisexual orientation. While families may be aware of a 'special friendship', they are usually unaware of the full expression, shared physically, mentally and socially. It is essential for all concerned to help the family and others to understand the uniqueness and the validity of this loving co-creative relationship.

While stress has been laid on the problems experienced by members of the gay community, this should not lessen our concern for others, for instance bisexual people, who are not wholly gay. Nor should we forget the drug abusers who are infected through the use of each other's dirty needles and syringes. Of equal importance are babies infected through their mother's bloodstream or breast feeding; also those infected with non-heat-treated blood products. Each one of these groups has need of pastoral care that is unique to each. Each too has families, partners and friends who need support.

'Worship cares for us'

The minister is expected to be with, to pray with and to serve sacramentally the sick, the dying, the bereaved and all who care for them – unconditionally according to their wishes.

Today it is increasingly accepted that, for the most part, isolation is unnecessary except where it is needed to protect the health of the person infected. Therefore, it is right that we should offer all the sacraments requested by this person as we would to anyone else in the hospital ward or at home. These include baptism, confirmation, reconciliation, eucharist, anointing and rites for releasing the person into the greater life.

I have found the four sacraments most asked for are laying-on of hands, anointing, reconciliation and eucharist. The patient may ask for each in his or her own time. We are not there to convert him or her. We are simply there to respond to his or her needs of the moment.

This means that our prayers and reading within or outside the communion service, whether in the ward, the hospital chapel or at home, demand that we be sensitive to the physical, mental and social sufferings of the person who is our concern. Thus, to read a passage or to offer prayers that are clearly related to sin is to increase his or her mental and physical suffering which will in turn increase a depression of his or her immune system, already severely damaged by HIV viral infection.

Reconciliation is often sought, although not usually in the formal manner. What is not needed is judgement or any sort of moralising. This is certainly not the time to express one's own anxieties and fears about different sexual activities or lifestyles. Instead what is of value is the concerned presence of another human being, one who is unafraid of being vulnerable, unafraid of expressing compassionate care in the holding of the hand, in the embrace and in the offering of a kiss. All are symbols of assurance, acceptance and a continuing inclusion in the family, in the community of lovers. This confirms for the sufferer what he or she really wants to know and needs to feel deep within: that he or she is wholly acceptable in his or her illness.

I want to stress again that this person, like myself, is created in the image of God – a God not obliterated by HIV infection, ARC or AIDS. As I have said before, so much of this will depend on how at ease we are with our own unique gift of sexuality and our own willingness to give and to receive affection. In truth, we have to ask ourselves as ministers: 'Have we the courage of faith to illuminate the Gospel of compassionate loving after the manner of Jesus Christ, our mutual brother, who is also infected with all the viruses and wounds of God's people?'

HIV infection and the chalice

It is important for us to accept that, as far as medical and scientific evidence is concerned, there is *no* reason at all to fear that the sharing of the common communion chalice will contribute to the spread of the AIDS virus. This is because the alcohol in the eucharistic wine has a certain disinfectant effect, even more so if the chalice is silver- or gold-plated.

There is *no* known case of anyone being infected orally via the chalice. It appears that saliva contains enzymes which inhibit the AIDS virus. Research continues to show that the sharing of common vessels for eating and drinking has played no role in the spread of the virus.

The advice given to our two archbishops has convinced

them that fears of infection are groundless. For those who are still anxious, two courses of action can be offered. The communicant can either receive communion in one kind only, i.e. the wafer or bread, or by intinction, i.e. retaining the consecrated bread until it can be dipped in the consecrated wine.

Those who are infected with HIV very often experience a great sense of rejection and isolation. Pastoral care demands that we should not be another source of this rejection and isolation by demanding that they either receive in one kind or by intinction or that they should refrain altogether from taking communion though being present with those who are.

There is some confusion about the wiping of the chalice after each communion. Some maintain that this reduces risk, others that it might increase it slightly unless one were to change the purificator after each communicant.

The virus is known to be fragile in the sense that it requires the right sort of physical environment – warm bodily fluids – if it is to survive and be transmitted. Obviously these conditions are not present when communicants receive from the chalice, even though it is true that the saliva of some infected patients has been found to contain the virus. To my knowledge, those I know who are seriously ill with the infection are more fearful of infecting others than we should be of being infected. The truth is that there is no record of anyone having been infected in this way with this virus or any other through the centuries. In accepting this truth our fears will dissolve and we shall be free to drink from the common chalice as a sign of our communion not only with Christ but also with each other, especially the person living with HIV infection, ARC or AIDS. This act will assure the person that he or she is a member of the Christian family because the eucharistic action is the centre of life and, in the breaking of bread and drinking from the shared cup, we all recognise our membership in the Christian community. The communion is offered with the compassion of Christ, the continuing suffering Christ, who is also suffering from HIV infection. Only our own personal fears will prevent us from offering the cup of unconditional love. Such fears, which are as real to ministers as anyone else, will only be removed through education and an understanding of the hidden fear behind the fears voiced.

The minister as the enabler

Christian and other friends who attempt to offer basic care should respect the person's need for privacy without ignoring his or her need for physical and emotional contact. They must sense when help is needed in dealing with everyday practical problems and know how to make the person feel welcome in their homes and encourage him or her in social activities. It is obviously essential to help out with those tasks that the person finds too difficult, but it must be done in such a way that the person is not made to feel useless and unwanted.

The carer recognises the 'personhood' of the sufferer and treats him or her as a real friend that he or she is proud to know and be with. The carer is warm and treats the person with respect and keeps confidential whatever personal information the sufferer and those who suffer with him or her wish to share. The carer is sensitive to special days and dates in the sufferer's own calendar and what these may mean. He or she is attentive to daily needs and demonstrates this by small acts of kindness, helping in the house, shopping, going to the launderette, mending clothes, changing library books or videos. The sensitive carer will also be aware of the sufferer's need to help the carer whose needs he or she will often recognise before the carer does. Vulnerability attracts vulnerability, as care attracts care. Shared caring is mutual caring according to the abilities of each person.

The minister, or other carers, should not become the centre, the focal point, of the care network, realising that no one person can care co-creatively for every need without support, personal and corporate.

With such support we can face the sufferer and those who are with him or her knowing that we do not shock easily and that we are able to accept human feelings (different as they are in each person) and are not embarrassed by tears or anger. We can be warm and affectionate, are able to touch with the embrace of care and to help the person recognise the new strengths that are emerging out of the pain of the infection. We can show that we recognise that growth is occurring and are able to accompany the person through this period of suffering. We are able to acknowledge to him or her and to others that we all share the rich gift of our humanness and to recognise and respect where he or she 'is at' at any one time during the worst of the illness. We are able to have a genuine respect for the person's sense of determination and at all times to treat him or her as an adult who can, in most instances, make his or her own decisions. We regard them as persons who are attempting to understand what they are really saying when they express feelings of fear, of hate, of particular sexual yearnings and fantasies. We understand that he or she is capable of being faithful to commitments and promises.

Those of us in the caring ministry will only be able to be empathetic if we have first listened to and become empathetic with ourselves. Care of self encourages care of others according to their needs and their desires. We can only come close to the sufferer and allow him or her to come close to us if we are both prepared to risk an honest sharing of ourselves, that we might become friends within the space of co-creative healing between us. This sharing occurs when we accept each other just as we are, with all our weaknesses and all our strengths, which in reality are one and the same.

We shall fulfil the request of Peter and others who are living with the HIV infection if we live as carers who are responding to our basic responsibilities to 'body forth' the Christian tradition of compassion. The norms of a sound theological reflection provide us with a framework in which to examine realistic ways and means of responding to the mutuality of our needs. This will only occur if we take time *to be, to listen* and *to hear* ourselves into the mystery, the uniqueness, of each person with whom we are concerned.

This meditative statement sums up for me the mystery of 'attentive listening', so essential if we are to hear the other person.

The one who listens attentively
   is the one who obeys,
   is the one who loves.

The one who listens attentively
  is the one prepared
  to stand
  face to face with God,
  face to face to the other person
  face to face with one's self
  and there
  find one's self
  face to face with Love.
The one who listens attentively
  is the one who obeys,
  is the one who loves Love.

It is crucial for us all to realise the truth, that the measure of our hearing is the measure of our listening. Equally the measure of our prayer is the true measure of the mutuality of our caring for and through each other.

10

Ethical and Moral Perspectives

For the Christian there can be no other ethic than that of love. This is the activity of encouraging the care and growth not only of oneself, but also of all others. I love myself that I may all the more be freed to love another into reaching his or her fullest potential. Love is for the nurturing of each other into a fullness of life that is worth living and dying for.

In sharing with you some thoughts on the ethics of pastoral care, I am not concerned with making moral judgements, but rather with our ability to be compassionate in our caring and to offer practical help, or to obtain such help that we may not be able to offer personally. The prime requisite of this help, I believe, is that we have a realistic awareness of who we are as persons, and of our ability to offer pastoral care of a non-judgemental nature and to accept that moralising is not appropriate in *any* illness.

To begin, we must be aware of our own falling short of the mark of perfection, our own sinfulness if you like, especially as we are all involved in the systemic weaknesses of the community. These weaknesses include oppression, racism, poverty, bigotry, fear, indifference, inhospitality, homophobia and various forms of addiction.

The ethical demand of our involvement in pastoral care is that of compassion. In the context of this ethic we must be aware of the dangers of drawing on theology to make quick and easy judgements. In so doing, we shall avoid the 'wrath of God' statements. AIDS is a viral infection, not a moral one, and it is not meant to be a test of our personal hang-ups and moral beliefs. We minister because the person is ill through the activity of a deadly virus working its bodily havoc. 'The molecular equivalent of the nuclear bomb' was how someone suffering 'Full-blown AIDS' expressed it to me.

To argue that AIDS is God's punishment on homosexuals and others is illogical and morally repugnant. The 'wrath of God' theory regarding this viral infection discloses more about the attitudes of those who hold it than it does about the nature of God's understanding and total acceptance of 'the person' of the sufferer. It is only from within the love ethic that we are made strong enough to refute such statements from whatever source they emanate. We do so in the awareness that such statements do not have sufficient biblical justification and are contrary to the teachings of Jesus, who saw through people's outer sicknesses, both mental and physical, to the whole person within who has been created in God's image.

I suggest that our pastoral concern is better directed towards the quality of life of the person living with the HIV infection rather than issues of sexual orientation and activities. Any of us who have ever tried to understand another's sexual orientation will realise it is something no one actually chooses. Our identity is what matters and we should accept the person who presents us with the truth of his or her identity *as a person*.

For me the basic ethic of the Church is to love non-judgementally. As ministers we have a moral responsibility to be the advocates of all sufferers, to be alongside the person of our concern. Equally, we have the responsibility to educate, to offer the same kind of care that we would offer to any other person who is ill, whatever the cause, as we realise that a bacteria or a virus is non-moral and as such does not raise moral or ethical problems.

I believe, as does Janet Morley, that the Church has a moral responsibility *not* to use the HIV infection to reclaim the age-old virtue of chastity

which may well reinforce the negative and distorted aspects of Christian teaching, rather than redeeming what is positive and life enhancing.

We should note that when chastity is produced as a solution to the threat of AIDS, we have shifted the meaning away from the area of moral choice and are describing behaviour that is simply prudent. To suggest (as the BSR report does [Board for Social Responsibility, AIDS – some guidelines for pastoral care, 1986]) that it would be better to recommend chastity than condoms because the latter are not 100% reliable, is to propose chastity not as a positive goal for life but simply as the most effective means of avoiding this kind of death.

Of course, people need to be warned about the precise risk and danger, both to their own life and that of others, but to confuse such a warning with moral guidance is to use the spectre of AIDS rather in the way the threat of hellfire used to be evoked. Again, moral teaching backed up by fear may be more or less what people expect of the Church, but is this really the whole extent of what the Christian tradition has to offer?

It is the Church's role to teach by example the positive aspects of celibacy, alongside the positive aspects of a monogamous relationship, irrespective of the sexual orientation of that relationship. The Church has a moral responsibility to re-examine its attitudes towards the God-given gift of sexuality and I believe that the onset of AIDS will force the Church to do so if it is to remain credible in its pronouncements regarding this viral infection.*

In our honest facing-up to the ethical and moral issues regarding AIDS, we need to remember the Archbishop of York's statement.

The world faces a medical crisis. But it is also a moral crisis. It is not simply a crisis of sexual morality, though restrained sexual behaviour is going to be increasingly important for the foreseeable future. The heart of the moral crisis is whether compassion and sensitivity and restraint towards one another can overcome fear, can encourage lifestyles which limit the spread of the disease, and can enable those infected by it to retain their dignity, and to

* Janet Morley, 'Redeeming Asceticism', *The Way*, vol. 27, no. 3 (July 1987).

die knowing that they are upheld in faith and hope and love.

How the churches emerge from this crisis is going to be a great test of our faithfulness to the gospel of the cross and resurrection.*

As Paul Clarke warns:

The search for scapegoats is both pointless and potentially harmful, possibly more harmful than the disease itself. Those who are bent on searching for scapegoats and who adopt dogmatic and/or bigoted viewpoints may well prove to be a public health hazard far greater than AIDS itself.†

The moral problem is not one of apportioning blame but of showing the care of compassion. We must not forget that the cause of this infection is a virus which is spread through types of activity that are not its cause. This is why we can say that AIDS is not just *our* problem or *their* problem. It is not *only* a national problem but an international problem on an ever-increasing scale. Unless we, the Church, tackle this problem internationally, millions of our brothers and sisters throughout the world will die and so will the Body of Christ.

Peter Jenkins describes AIDS as 'perhaps the greatest peacetime challenge to the governments in our time'. Equally, I believe, it is one of the greatest challenges to the compassion that faces the Christian and all others who profess to care. There is no doubt that this viral infection has the potential for releasing the best and the worst in people.

The ethical demands of our ministry must begin with the awareness that we are caring for a person with a personal experience that is unique to that person; while he or she is *inside* the experience, we are *outside* it. The HIV infection, like any other life-threatening infection, has a spiritual dimension arising out of a traumatic experience of knowing that one is infected and may die as a result.

There is no doubt that we must battle not only for those living with the infection, but also their partners, families and friends – and for ourselves that we do not fall victim, through

* Diocesan leaflet, January 1987.
† *Sunday Times*, 9 November 1986.

87

fear, to the withholding of compassion, because we have lost sight of the qualities we hold most dear as Christians, like friendship and stability of purpose.

Somehow, through all this suffering, we must have the courage of faith to offer the vital elixir of realism, hope and love. Our purpose alongside the person is to encourage a quality of relationship that is rich in the mutuality of concerned care. Our responsibility is to recognise the undeniable fact that morality must not be linked to this viral infection: all diseases in themselves are non-moral. It is crucial that the Church keeps itself well informed of the real facts about AIDS. It has a moral duty to communicate this information as a practical way of demonstrating its concerned care, through its natural network of clubs, groups, the laity and its ordained and professed leaders. It is very important that its practical work is strengthened through prayer and meditation and through its liturgies for all who are suffering and living with the illness and those who are suffering alongside them.

The Christ-like ministry is that of compassionate concern. It is also a challenge to us individually and collectively as members of the Church of God, the Church of love, to embrace lovingly all who are suffering the ravages of this human immunodeficiency disease. The pastoral ethic arises out of the prime ethic of love. For the Christian, it surpasses all others.

The *Ad Clerum* from the Bishops of London Diocese, April 1987, sums up these ethical issues for us:

> As Christians, our first responsibility to people who suffer from AIDS or who are infected with the AIDS virus, is to give them the response we owe to anyone who is sick. In visiting and caring for the sick, we are ministering to the Lord himself (Matthew 25:40). Furthermore, if we belong to Christ and are entrusted with a share in his ministry, this includes touching those whom society treats as untouchable, and embracing those whom society isolates. We must, therefore, not only support all who are engaged in the professional care of AIDS sufferers; we must also be ready to offer our own practical help to those who need it.

For instance, by doing the shopping, washing, cooking or cleaning for people who have become too weak to do it themselves. Christians also have a duty to resist ignorance and fear. This involves remedying their own ignorance and facing their own fears.

Safer sex

For those *not* infected with the virus, their ethical and moral responsibility, not only towards others but also towards themselves and the whole of society, is to practice safer sex. Certainly the most effective way to prevent the spread of this virus is to avoid all risky sexual activities, irrespective of one's sexual orientation. We all have an obligation to life, to live it co-creatively and to keep ourselves in reasonably good health. Therefore, anything done carelessly in the passion of the moment which prevents this, may lead to severely damaged health or death. Such action would be irresponsible. For the person already infected, the ethical and moral responsibility is even more compelling, especially that of avoiding infecting others. The tension that this will cause between personal freedom and public health will be solved only by making difficult choices. It is important to remember that a basic condition of life is making choices. It is crucial that there be a right balance of care between the needs, including the sexual needs, of the infected person and not only the health care of the partner but also the interests of public health generally.

AIDS is a natural killer in the sense that man did not invent the virus itself. It has been called a 'disease of options', of 'choices for consenting adults'. As such it would be better, therefore, to educate for a change from high risk practices to low risk practices. Obviously, it is not an infection of consenting adults or others where rape is concerned.

Increasingly, one must be worried for the teenagers who, as they become sexually aware of themselves, will, as we did, experiment and may have several partners before moving into a co-creative relationship. It is crucial that parents, teachers and students are told, non-hysterically, about this sexually transmitted disease in the hope that they may pass on the facts to their children and pupils, from the age of twelve upwards, within the context of teaching about the whole spectrum of sexuality.

There is much talk of isolation for those who are infected with the virus. This would not only be impractical when one considers the thousands who are infected not only in this country but also throughout the world. It would also be prohibitive costwise. In addition, it would have a negative effect on those who are actually suffering because their immune systems are no longer a fertile breeding ground for the virus. It is the unidentified infected who do not practice 'safer sex' who are the source of infection to their sexual partners and to drug users who share needles as part of their fixing ritual.

In all this confusion, we need to be aware that, while research is absolutely essential, it also poses certain dangers for the person involved. These dangers include the possible loss of the individual's rights of protection againt any unjustifiable harm and of all guarantees of privacy and the strict maintenance of confidentiality. We must see HIV infection as contrary to the general trend in modern medicine and our belief in medicine's potential to cure, if not heal, all manner of diseases, be they physical, mental, social or spiritual. To a society brought up on the idea that disease is diminishing, we are shattered at the appearance of a virulent, and yet intractable, new disease that is socially unacceptable.

The ethical and moral problems created by this infection force us to recognise the weaknesses and strengths of our own attitudes.

To test or not to test

One of the moral issues connected with the HIV infection is that of antibody testing, especially when a positive result does not guarantee the eventual development of ARC/AIDS or other disorders of the immune system. Conversely, a negative result is not definitive.

T. H. Murray and G. M. Aumann in their chapter 'Ethical issues in AIDS' sum up the moral issues by saying that responsible screening programmes must ask and satisfactorily answer five questions:

1 For whom is the testing being done – the person tested (first-person benefit) or others (third-person)? Other than informing those who wish to know, HTLV-III/LAV testing today confers few benefits on the person tested. Justifications are usually made in terms of benefit to third parties.

2 Is testing voluntary or mandatory? Voluntary testing raises few moral problems. Most of the difficult questions come with mandatory testing.

3 What will be done with the information? What acceptable social goals can be achieved through screening? At what ethical and economic costs? The history of genetic screening is rife with cases where no thought was given to this question.

4 Will this screening program permit us to reach the desired goal? What are the acceptable realistic goals? Will this program achieve them?

5 Is this the least intrusive and restrictive means to the goal? It is not enough to reach the goal if we could have done so with less harm.*

Testing will only be acceptable if those found to be antibody positive are given statutory assurances that they will not be discriminated against in their health and social care needs; in the obtaining of life insurance, mortgages and long-term bank or other loans; in their places of work; and in their social activities and within society generally.

All blood in the UK is now tested for HIV antibodies. If they are detected in the donor's blood, it is again tested. If the finding is confirmed, the donor is contacted and counselled. All donors sign a form agreeing to his or her blood being tested for HIV.

Health and care personnel

Professional and other reaction to those suffering and working within this area of need has generally been good, although

* T. H. Murray and G. M. Aumann, in Gong and Rudnick (Eds), *AIDS: facts and issues* (Rutgers University Press, 1986).

there are some who have refused point blank to have anything to do with those who are HIV infected and their carers. This is usually due to their own inner insecurity and fears nourished through ignorance. Even though they may have chosen to be carers, the moral force of a professional commitment means nothing if it applies only to caring with and for those to whom it appears to be safe to offer one's services. It is crucial that health and other care personnel recognise that in their response to AIDS the public will see how deep a moral commitment doctors, nurses, social workers and ministers have actually made.

It is important for health care workers and others to recognise that attitudes to the onslaught of this disease are causing many changes that are undoubtedly detrimental to those living with the infection, at whatever stage. Their ongoing care can be blocked because life and health insurances are made more difficult, if not near impossible, to obtain. Life insurance companies are beginning to include in the original questionnaire questions like 'Have you ever been involved in blood-testing for AIDS or hepatitis?' Similar considerations apply to mortgages and any other loans which require life cover. Private health care too is now imposing its own rules. Some schemes stipulate a five-year period for new members who join during which benefits for the care of AIDS related conditions and AIDS itself will not be paid.

Health and social care costs will rocket as all groups of medical, nursing and social care personnel are retrained in an effort to change attitudes of fear and the oppression of blame. As more and more people succomb to the ravages of the disease the bill will rise.

The environment of society

There is a very real danger that, as the panic passes, AIDS may become either a bore, and therefore an acceptable risk, or a stimulus to various forms of official and unofficial repression. Alongside this danger, there are those who are making political, economic, social and religious capital out of AIDS, while the suffering continues, because those infected are being discarded as *non-persons*, a burden to society that it is unwilling to bear.

Ethically and morally we need to recognise that every member of the community (locally, nationally and internationally) deserves to be protected from any communicable disease including that of fear. This is a basic human right. Everyone is entitled to equal consideration and respect.

Many suffering from this viral infection do not fit the medical and nursing models which label them 'patients' when in fact, for the most part, they are not ill enough to be described in that way. It is true that AIDS is a clinical problem, but it is also a *social* problem with clinical manifestations. Surely what we must look for is a balanced social solution in which human well-being is the norm.

Dr Paul Clarke argues* that 'it is not . . . beyond the bounds of conceivability that mankind is, unintentionally, both the author of the virus and of its development into epidemic form'. He puts forward a very strong case, 'namely that the structural changes in society had been of such an order that society's own immune defences are suppressed. While the AIDS virus is an opportunistic infection of the human body, "AIDS the Syndrome" can be regarded as an opportunistic infection of the lowered immune system of the social structure itself.' Paul Clarke suggests that any lasting cure requires not only removing the cause but also the reconstruction of the social structure in such a way that its immune system is not further suppressed, but revitalised.

Government ministers will admit that there is a moral dimension to the problem but are cautious in approaching that dimension directly, 'realising that moral preaching is not the business of government and will hardly change current attitudes. Preaching will merely harden these attitudes or even produce a backlash which will alienate the very people that need to be reached . . .'†

Certainly governments are not there to preach hellfire and brimstone (for that matter, neither is the Church). However, governments and the Church, while they should not moralise,

---

* Paul A. B. Clarke, *AIDS: Medicine, Politics and Society* (Lester Crook Academic, 1988).
† ibid.

can provide a framework within which ethical and moral debates of a serious nature could and must take place. It seems to me that part of that moral and ethical ground should include information on what does and does not constitute a co-creative relationship.

It is crucial that we accept the fact that the moral issue is not one of blame but of compassion and care. Paul Clarke argues* that

> all issues of blame and castigation need to be set aside in favour of the cohesive power of care. Only in this way can the potential divisiveness of this potential plague be not only overcome but also transcended, leaving no doubt in its wake many casualties but also many individual and collective victories; that and not the cesspit of blame is the moral challenge; it is also the harder challenge and its sheer difficulty is the no doubt real, and ultimately cowardly, reason behind the tendency to seek for scapegoats . . . There is a real danger of leper colony mentality, of an 'us-them' attitude developing when and if the disease reaches noticeable proportions.

Paul Clarke points out that the greatest challenge of all for society will be how to bring out the best in people, sufferer and carer alike. This means that the campaign against AFRAIDS must begin now before fear sets in and produces minds so closed that there will be no way to unlock and enter those closed minds. If this challenge is approached with care, caution and compassion, then the problem of bringing the pragmatic and moral approaches together will not only be surmountable, it will be salutory and will offer the best hope of leaving for the future a reasonable legacy that we and future generations can live with.

Murray and Aumann have identified for us at least four groups who have special moral responsibilities with respect to AIDS:

---

* Paul A. B. Clarke, *Aids: the political and social implications of an evolutionary advantageous retrovirus*, Memorandum to the Social Services Committee of the House of Commons on an Inquiry into Problems Associated with AIDS, no. A92.

First, health professionals, particularly physicians and nurses, have the same duty to treat AIDS patients and respect their right to confidentiality as they have toward all other patients. The risk of contracting AIDS in the line of duty appears to be highly exaggerated, but, even if not, the obligation would still exist. *Second*, scientists doing research on AIDS have an especially strong obligation to respect personal confidentiality. Failure to fulfil this obligation may both invalidate present research and make it more difficult to gain the confidence of subjects for future research. *Third*, people infected by the AIDS virus have a moral responsibility to take reasonable precautions to protect their own health and the health of others, which may mean modifying sexual behaviour and refraining from donating blood. *Fourth*, society has the same obligation to people with AIDS as it has to others who need assistance in the maintenance of health and treatment of illness. Society must take great care in fashioning public policies towards AIDS to assure that those policies are scientifically well informed and ethically acceptable.*

We shall only be able to live out our moral responsibilities with respect to this viral infection if we rethink honestly our social, moral and ethical values. This means being courageous enough to change what must be changed and to rejoice at what need not be changed.

* Murray and Aumann, op. cit.

11

The Church's Involvement

Costing not less then everything

Ministry

Basically, there are *no* areas where the specific gifts of each member of the Church could not be involved in ministering both to those living and suffering with the HIV infection and to those who are suffering alongside them.

Our first responsibility is to transcend the debate about how God views the sexual activities of all his people, be they hetero-, bi- or homo-sexual in orientation. We do this by recognising and accepting the fact that a disease itself has nothing to do with a person's sexual orientation. We also do it by acknowledging that all who are living with and suffering from this viral infection (however it has been contracted) remain sons and daughters of God who, as our ultimate lover, does not know how to cast out his beloved people. There is no way in which the Church can offer compassionate care unless we Christians, as individuals, empty our minds of any lingering suspicion that God may be using this infection as a punishment. The HIV infection is certainly challenging the Church to look objectively at the whole God-given gift of sexuality and the various co-creative ways of offering this gift one to another.

As Christians, our basic vocational responsibility is to be lovers of all God's people. Anyone who loves can be a *minister of presence* to the totalness of those in need of the friendship of acceptance (virus and all), a friendship that both authenticates them and shows them that they matter unconditionally. We ennoble each other when we are prepared to be the humanised embodiment of God's compassionate loving. We are 'to be as compassionate as your Father is compassionate'. We cannot be compassionate (the word means 'sorrow for the sufferings of another') unless we know the state of the heart of the person suffering. We minister best when we recognise that we are being ministered to by the love of Christ which was always mutual, just as it was always practical in meeting the real needs of the sufferer.

Unfortunately, at present, we minister knowing that, in many instances, the individual living with the infection will not walk into his or her local church for help. For so many, the Church has rejected them because of their sexual orientation.

As ministering carers, we need to encourage the development of a 'charter for care' (similar to the one passed at the 1986 General Convention of the Episcopal Church in the USA) for presentation and affirmation at the next Lambeth Conference, in 1988, i.e.

1 To offer compassionate care towards all who are living with the HIV infection, including their partners, families and friends.

2 To repudiate constantly any condemnation, rejection or judgement against those who are living with the viral infection.

3 To stress the crucial need for education and to be in the forefront of this first line of defence against infection.

4 To be with, to pray with, to remember liturgically and to serve sacramentally the sick, the dying, the bereaved and all who care with and for them.

The Church is expected to be a 'people's ministry' to all the peoples of God, and especially to the marginalised, the sick, the suffering and those who suffer with them. It is expected to support those involved in pre-bereavement and bereavement counselling. At all times we must respect the dignity and the confidentiality that will be demanded of us as trustees of faith, hope and love. We can enable each other, individually and collectively, to become part of a 'network' of 'listeners who hear' what is going on within and around the person of our concern. It is through attentive hearing that we are given clues as to how to educate co-creatively.

Education

The Churches are ideally positioned to encourage the collection and distribution of facts regarding the various stages and needs of those living with the disease. Through the mailing lists of the British Council of Churches, the National Synod, the Dioceses, the Methodist Conference and other similar bodies, the Churches can become partners in education with others in a joint preparation of study days, information packs, education programmes stressing the medical and social facts, awareness and understanding of the sexual spectrum, ethical and moral problems, listening and counselling training, home-care training, buddy training and liturgical training.

The Church must not be afraid to become involved in national and international discussion via the mass media. This will, I hope, encourage us all (locally, nationally and internationally) to face up to the health, social, economic, political, ethical and religious issues in all their interdependent manifestations.

The Church must recognise and welcome as colleagues in all our education and training programmes those living with the infection. Their insights and knowledge will surpass ours because, as I have emphasised before, each such person is living *inside* and we are living *outside* the infection.

Advocacy

The Church has a definite function of advocacy on behalf of *all* sufferers, whatever the nature or source of their life-threatening illness, against any form of discrimination in connection with health, social and home-care needs, housing accommodation, employment security, pensions, mortgages and long-term loans. We should not only be active in fund-raising schemes (local, national and international), but also encouraging the parish, the deanery, the diocese and the central Church to help establish the various services which will be required and to pay key salaries in this specialised vocational area of care.

The Church should advocate the full support of the partner of the infected person whatever the co-creative nature of their relationship and recognise the validity of same-sex partnerships so often unsupported by the Church and by others.

The Church must advocate 'safer sex' and be aware of the different sexual needs and energies of all those who are sexually active. Ministers need to accept that sexual activity as a procreative or co-creative function should be encouraged. It is their responsibility to help educate people to practise 'safer sex'. We must also be aware that most of those at the height of their sexual drives and needs are young people who are often not prepared (as many of us were not) to be limited to one partner, whatever their sexual orientation. It follows therefore that we have a responsibility to encourage the use of condoms, not to prevent procreation but rather to prevent death. A judgemental or moralising stance is of no help, although this does not mean to say that ministers and other carers approve of any sexual activity which abuses or dehumanises the other person or indeed oneself. Where it is known that a particular lifestyle has dangerous connotations, the minister should encourage a change and support the person in making it, although, once again, the person will not be helped if the minister takes a judgemental or moralising stance.

The Church must advocate flexibility when choosing between the different types of home and hospice care available. The person living with and through the experience of being infected with the virus should be encouraged to share in deciding what practical support he or she needs, rather than be forced to accept our own idea of what is best. This sensitive approach is particularly important between bouts of hospitalisation, and such caring, supported by medical, nursing and social work advisers, can be genuinely positive and fruitful for all involved. With such understanding, we can together enable the person with ARC/AIDS to live as fully as possible within the various limitations set by the disease, and in such a way that the fear of dying gives way to a notion of the dignity of dying.

I must stress again that the Church must be an advocate, *and be seen to be so*, of all who are infected or caught up in the different ramifications of this disease.

AIDS – a challenge to the Church

AIDS is a challenge to our compassion, if we are to be faithful to Jesus, who called and appointed us to follow his example in our attitude towards our brothers and sisters. To do this, we have no alternative but to embrace the unique personhood of every sufferer and of those who suffer with them. This is the work of God-in-Christ and of Christ-in-us-all. This is the work of love's compassionate endeavouring towards all who suffer, whatever the form of suffering, and those who suffer with them.

We must be humble enough to allow those living with the virus to minister to us through their suffering. It is their suffering that releases the mutuality of our compassion, one to another. This is in the awareness that, if one member suffers, we all suffer; that if one member has AIDS, we all have AIDS. For the Christian this is a reminder that the Church, as the body of Christ, also has AIDS. This is why Jesus can say 'inasmuch as you have done it unto one of these, the least of these my brothers [and my sisters], you have done it to me', as we each in our way fulfil the overwhelming need of practical Christian caring for all who are ill, suffering or dying from this infection. Their suffering is no more the 'will of God' than it is the will of God that anyone should die of cancer, or should die in agony after a car crash.

The Christian is expected to be 'infected', through the pains of doubt, with *'Faith, Hope and Love, and the greatest of all these is Love'*. This will release the innate healing energies lying dormant within every person. We are expected to be unafraid of recognising the suffering and loving Jesus, and ourselves, in the person of the sufferer.

An eastern Staretz (spiritual soul-friend), Father Silouhan, puts it very simply: 'My brother, my sister is my life.' In saying this, he reminds us of the basic truths of the Gospel, that the other person is my, is our, brother, sister, who is my and your life. When we accept this fact and act accordingly, there is a real chance of healing taking place, whether towards a fullness of life in this dimension of our being or in that next life which is beyond our comprehension.

We achieve this fullness, whether we are sufferers or non-sufferers, by being involved in the mystery of shared enabling, nourished as we are through the compassion of love's endeavouring for all God's people and ourselves. Our basic vocational responsibility as Christians is to serve without counting the cost of our expenditure of *love's compassion*. Only a healthy network of love will release the much needed epidemic of compassion towards all who suffer.

Father Bernard Lynch when asked 'How does one begin the journey of shared compassion?' had this to say:

It happens by people like you and me reaching out to one another, not with judgement but with an openness that is love. To be open to someone is to become that person; a person becomes what they are open to. For us to be open as Christians is to be open to the infinite possibilities of an infinitely loving God. Literally the skies are the limit. We are called not into a spirit of slavery but into a spirit of freedom. We are God's gay and non-gay daughters and sons. Our Daddy is King – what more could you ask?*

In this, he is reminding us that the only co-creative response to the HIV infection is a passionate desire to be a channel of healing, as was and is Jesus.

Any other posture is an insult to Jesus and is totally unworthy of the name 'Christian'. The sufferer, whatever the nature of the suffering, is saying like him, 'I thirst for Love'. Have we the courage of faith to share the cup of love not only with those like ourselves but also with others? That is the question. We are expected to clothe with love those who are naked of love.

The Church, through the epidemic of HIV infection, is being called into initiating what might be called 'an epidemic of compassion', nurtured through compassionate action and empathetic counselling. Any ministry to those affected by the

* Interviewed on the Late, Late Show, 3 April 1987; quoted in *Out*, no. 12.

different stages of this infection has a dual function: that of caring not only for those who are actually living and suffering with the infection, but also for those whose alienation, whether self-imposed or otherwise, is part of the epidemic of AIDS. The Church must do all in its power to prevent the epidemic of alienation that the AIDS diagnosis could bring, leaving us standing as before a huge chasm of fear. On the one side is the person suffering the effects of this infection, who so often stands alone and separated from the other world that was his life, his selected family and friends. On the other side, threateningly, can be unenlightened society, if we allow it. For the gay person and others, alienation is so often the result of legal, medical, social and religious oppression.

So many gay people have been ostracised by the Church that they are unlikely to look to it as to a caring parent, for the compassionate love God bears towards his vulnerable people. For many, the judgement of the Church is the judgement of God. It is because of this that most are forced to choose between the gift of his or her particular sexual orientation and his or her particular spirituality.

The Church needs to allow itself to be healed of its fears of the gift of sexuality and to recognise in this gift the many ways of expressing it co-creatively. Once it has the courage of faith to do this, then it will be able to repent of the sin of alienation which it has engendered. This will only occur through an openly honest acknowledgement and understanding of why and how its actions, and inactions, have contributed to the pain of alienation for so many from the Church of God. Until the Church is recognised as a welcoming place for all persons, gay and otherwise, its inherent healing ministry of compassionate loving will be minimised and it will be in no kind of reconciling position to proclaim the Good News of the 'Gospel of Love'. Neither will it have the courage of faith to offer the boundary-breaking love of Jesus to the poor and the lepers of today. All that those who should be in our care are asking for is the acceptance of love and an affirmation of their unlimited potential for growth into life. They wish to be enabled to die with the dignity of love, when this is the only way forward, through a kind of loving that is liberating enough to allow us to share mutually

102

in one another's brokenness, as wounded healers, in a broken world. As we nourish each other with the energising food of reconciling love, we will be able to fulfil and be the Gospel within the AIDS crisis that challenges the Church in deed and in truth. Let us take the following four statements to heart:

- The Christian Gospel lays before us a clear imperative of compassion and caring. This tradition, as well as sound theological reflection, provides us with a framework in which to examine and find ways of responding to people's needs.
- In the mysteries of life and death we encounter God. This encounter calls us to trust, hope and awe, rather than paralysis and immobilisation. Those we cannot cure we can support and sustain in solidarity: 'I was hungry – thirsty – a stranger – naked – sick – imprisoned – and you fed – clothed – took care – visited (Matthew 25).
- The AIDS crisis challenges us to be the Church in deed and in truth: to be the Church as a healing community. AIDS is heartbreaking and challenges the Churches to break their own hearts, to repent of inactivity and of rigid moralisms. Since AIDS cuts across race, class, gender, age, sexual orientation and sexual expression, it challenges our fears and exclusions. The healing community itself will need to be healed by the forgiveness of Christ.
- The people of God can be the family that embraces and sustains those who are sick with AIDS or AIDS related conditions, caring for the sister, brother or child without barriers, exclusion, hostility or rejection.

As ministers and care offerers:

We are to look into the eyes of the sufferer and see there the grief, fear, pleading, courage, anger, resignation, hope: how can you not show compassion? Will this new disease bring forth in us a new tenderness, a willingness to pay the price of healing that is to suffer with, especially with those we are tempted to despise? That was the whole point of the parable of the Good Samaritan. The correct lawyer was given the example of one who, as a good Jew of that time, he would most deeply despise, a Samaritan. Follow the example of those you reject. Being kind in a crisis is one thing – the whole situation is given a sharp challenge when you are shown up by someone you dislike for not doing enough. Let the ones without fault or failure do the condemning. Otherwise, give to each and all the respect that is the birthright of being human.

And being weak doesn't mean the end of our influence. Accepting that for now we may be a weak spot may mean that we can allow that powerless place to become the exact point through which mercy can flow into our lives and into the lives of those with whom we have to do. Sometimes it is the very obstacles that we cannot get rid of in ourselves that, accepted and pressed into gently, become the places where others find their healing. If they sense that we know deeply the trials of suffering and of dying, they will beat a path to our door, and we both may find a deeper healing, in a wondrously strange exchange. We shall have become 'priests' in the only sense of the word that matters, living at the centre of sacrifice, the utter giving upon which the world depends for everything.*

Quite clearly our first responsibility is to respond to the best of our individual and corporate abilities to the needs of 'the least of these my brothers [and sisters]' in every situation as we attempt to be the minister of Christ in today's suffering world, as together we find ourselves sharing the pain of AIDS. We are summoned by love to be love. 'This is my body, this is my blood', this is my loving embrace. Together we must share the pain of this viral infection unconditionally.

The General Synod of the Church of England debates AIDS

In the debate on AIDS at the General Synod on 10 November 1987, the Archbishop of Canterbury speaking on the report by the Board for Social Responsibility stated:

I hope this motion will be plainly accepted. More, I hope

---

* Jim Cotter, *What Price Healing in a Time of Epidemic?* (Cairns Publications, 1987).

this brief balanced and constructive report will be read and used by all of us in any way concerned with questions about AIDS.

However, I want to make it clear where I stand and where I think we should stand as a Church.

We affirm our traditional teaching and we ask for compassion. We welcome the initiatives being taken by Her Majesty's Government and others, but we insist that there are theological, moral and pastoral issues also to be taken up . . .

One of the first things human beings do when they are frightened is to look for someone to blame. A characteristic symptom of a plague is a witch-hunt. We have seen something of this with the AIDS plague. I believe it is based on bad theology. Disease is no respecter of virtue. Christians must have better ways of dealing with fear. We have no need to distance ourselves from those who are suffering. We should know that love casts out fear but not by dodging it. And when the fear includes shame, stigma and loneliness, that is also comprehended in the death which Christ died . . .

Secondly, we can say that the strength of the Christian Gospel is that it has something to say to people where they are. Now is the time that counts. Even if we think people have brought their troubles on their own heads, to say 'I told you so. You should never have got yourself into this mess' is about as far from Christianity as any utterance could be. We have to take the situation as it is and this means that we have to be ready to speak differently to different people. Some need warnings, some need information, some need comfort, some need practical help.

Can we be alert enough to provide what is needed when it is needed and not offer comfort to the complacent and judgement to the miserable? And can we be brave enough to accept the fact that whatever we offer we are likely to be misunderstood? Our comfort will lull the complacent and our judgement will distress the miserable . . .

Thirdly, our contribution has to be offered from humility as well as from confidence. First the humility to accept how much human effort is being made which Christians are called to affirm in this battle . . .

Christians down the centuries have always shared in the task of resisting disease and seeking ways of countering it. So we must support the urgent task of research and encourage those committed to it to continue the struggle to find the answers we need.

It is sometimes suggested that it is our duty in the Church to talk about chastity and fidelity, while it is the duty of public bodies to deal with the practical issues such as adequate contraceptive advice and the provision of clean needles for people who inject drugs. I have no hesitation in supporting the need to offer detailed down-to-earth practical advice.

But I want us to accept the major challenge. There is a responsibility on all of us to speak of what is required in our personal relations if this disease is to be brought under control. And the only safe way of preventing the spread of this disease in our society is through fidelity. That is what we mean by safe sex. Many have thought that the physical pleasure of sex can be divorced from its moral commitment. The price of that divorce is very high. If you try to love on a limited liability basis, you limit your ability to love at all. It is for these reasons that the Church upholds the idea of Christian marriage, life-long, exclusive and faithful as the only setting in which human sexuality can be responsibly and fully enjoyed. Our business is not to frighten people into good behaviour but to enable them to see human beings, both themselves and others, as children of God whose bodies are sacred, not disposable sex aids, and whose happiness lies in the sharing of a whole life, not in mere encounters in bed.

That is the Church's teaching: fidelity. Contrary to popular misconceptions, it applies to a lot more than sex. It is part of our vision of man as made in the image of God. In innumerable ways it is the duty of all of us to share with others the vision that has been given to us and to work out its implications for sex, as for all other aspects of life. We do this not just as bishops pontificating on platforms or priests sermonising in pulpits, but in the arguments we have in factory and office, the advice we give our own children at home, the teaching we give in schools, the way we answer the probing questions of students or members of youth clubs and, above all, in the way we lead our own lives.

I believe that challenge needs to be faced by everyone as we come to terms with the reality of AIDS. We are therefore quite right to press public bodies, education authorities and all concerned with the prevention of this disease to lay stress on the need for faithfulness and chastity. We ought to be able to present it with confidence, but also with humility for we have so often presented Christian social sexual ethics as a matter of dismal prohibitions or gone along with feeble permissiveness . . .

If we believe in the love of God as we have glimpsed it in Jesus, AIDS can have no final victory over us. The task of care, of fighting back and of learning new patterns of personal discipline can be full of hope for us and for our world.

The motion, passed overwhelmingly on a show of hands, was:

That this Synod, in the face of the serious threat posed by AIDS and affirming the Church's traditional teaching on chastity and fidelity in personal relationships:

- welcomes the concern reflected in the initiatives taken by Her Majesty's Government and statutory and voluntary bodies
- urges all members of the Church of England to respond with compassion and understanding to all those affected by AIDS
- requests the House of Bishops and the Board for Social Responsibility to continue to advise the Church on the theological, moral and pastoral issues involved.

Church of England members were urged by the General Synod of the Church to show compassion and understanding to *all* affected by AIDS and to have an unqualified care for those living with HIV infection. The primary responsibility of all its members was to show the face of love and to act with compassion according to need, not only towards all who are infected but equally to the partner, families and friends. We must seek to respond through informed understanding that will release us from the ignorance of fear.

The General Synod gave overwhelming approval to the Board for Social Responsibility's report 'AIDS'. In so doing, they agreed with the Board that this disease could not (no more than any other) be seen as God's judgement. Indeed, to believe so, is bad theology; it is not the theology of love but rather of fear. The debate about AIDS and judgement echoes the theological debate between the 'wrath of God' and the 'love of God'. To add guilt to AIDS because of a wish to be morally pious is downright sinful.

The Church must at all costs avoid 'making lepers' by heaping guilt not only on those infected by this viral infection but also on those associated with them. If the Church is to be the Church of God in Christ, then it has no alternative but physically, mentally and spiritually to hold hands and embrace all those who are living with this infection and all who suffer because of their association with the infected person.

It was suggested during the debate on AIDS 'that ecumenical, local task forces should be set up to co-ordinate work and liaise with organisations like the Terrence Higgins Trust'. It was also suggested that 'the Anglican Church should follow the example of the United Reformed Church in appointing a full-time adviser'.

During the past two years a number of diocesan guidelines on pastoral care has been published. Increasingly, Social Responsibility Officers of the different Diocesan Boards are spearheading educational conferences at all levels in their respective areas. Those who attend, laity, the ordained and the professed, are seeking informed information about the infection and its varying manifestations, to dispel fears and to suggest how persons affected can best be cared for.

Opportunity is now being given for people to examine their attitudes to lifestyles and sexual orientation different from their own and to examine their attitudes to dying and death. Also, more discussions are being led by those who are actually living with the virus, those who are caring for them and those who have been or who are being bereaved.

Christians of all denominations are being informed as to how they can realistically contribute to the ongoing care of those who are affected by the HIV infection. Increasingly, other denominations are becoming involved and, more often than not, as an ecumenical team. The Terrence Higgins Trust has an inter-faith team, in recognition of the fact that the virus is no respecter of the barriers of denomination.

In all this, we are reminded that we are all 'oned' to each other. We are all each other's life, each other's compassion, motivated by love, the absolute law of God in Christ, of God in and beyond all faiths. All of us need to remember that it is only the mystery of Love alone that is able to embrace, without any words, the suffering of anyone living with HIV infection and its consequences. The Church has called everyone to love all God's people and to accept that it has to work with and care for people with AIDS including all those who are at the sharp end, the 'burn-out' end, of the crisis.

The least you do unto one of these my brothers and sisters (our brothers and sisters), you do unto me (you do unto yourself).

A Litany of Reconciliation*

Almighty God, creator of life, sustainer of every good thing I know, my partner with me in the pain of this earth, hear my prayer as I am in the midst of separation and alienation from everything I know to be supportive, and healing, and true.

AIDS has caused me to feel separated from you. I say, 'Why me, what did I do to deserve this?' . . . Help me to remember that you do not punish your creation by bringing disease, but that you are Emmanuel, God with us. You are as close to me as my next breath.

AIDS has caused a separation between the body I knew and my body now. . . Help me to remember that I am more than my body and, while it pains me greatly to see what has happened to it, I am more than my body . . . I am part of you and you me.

AIDS has separated me from my family . . . Oh God help me and them to realise that I haven't changed, I'm still their child, our love for each other is your love for us . . . Help them overcome their fear, embarrassment and guilt . . . Their love brought me into this world . . . Help them share as much as possible with me.

AIDS has caused a separation between me and my friends; my friendships have been so important to me. They are especially important now . . . Help me oh God to recognise their fear, and help them to realise my increasing need for them to love in any way they can.

AIDS has separated me from my society, my work world and

* Author unknown.

my community . . . It pains me for them to see me differently now . . . Forgive them for allowing their ignorance of this disease and their fear to blind their judgements . . . Help me with my anger towards them.

AIDS has caused a separation between me and my Church . . . Help the Church restore its ministry to 'the least of these' by reaching out to me and others . . . Help them suspend their judgements and love me as they have before . . . Help me and them to realise that the Church is the Body of Christ . . . that separation and alienation wound the body.

God of my birth and God of my death, help me know you have been, you are, and you are to come . . . Amen

Prayer

Help us to accept the challenge of AIDS:
    To protect the healthy, calm the fearful;
    to offer courage to those in pain;
    to embrace the dying as they flow
        into love's unendingness;
    to console the bereaved;
    to support all those who attempt to care
        for the sick and the dying.

Enable us to offer our energies,
our imaginations,
and our trusting in the mysteries of love,
to be united with and through one another
in liberating each other
from fear of this disease.

We offer these thoughts and prayers
in the mystery of the loving
that can and does bear all our woundings,
whatever their source,
through the spirit of love's concern
for each and every person.   Amen

Glossary

AIDS (Acquired Immune Deficiency Syndrome)

A collection of illnesses that impair the body's ability to fight infection, making the body extremely susceptible to opportunistic infections. The definition of the syndrome also includes diagnosed affliction with certain opportunistic infections, such as Pneumocystis carinii pneumonia, or with certain cancers, such as Kaposi's sarcoma.

ADC (AIDS Dementia Complex)

Occurs when the HIV virus has passed through the blood-brain barrier, which usually 'filters' out substances in the blood which might damage the brain. Should this occur, then the person may suffer from memory loss and difficulty in walking and may require complete bodily and social care for the rest of his or her life.

Amyl nitrate

See 'Poppers'.

Antibodies

Any substance in the blood serum or other body fluids that destroys or neutralises bacteria, viruses or other harmful toxins that enter the body.

Antigens

Any substance which, when introduced into the body, causes the production of a specific antibody. The HIV virus is such a substance.

Antiviral

A type of substance that can destroy or weaken the pathogenic action of a virus. Antiviral drugs are being used experimentally against the AIDS virus.

ARC (AIDS Related Complex)

HIV has, by now, severely damaged the natural immune

113

system. The person is suffering from diarrhoea, excessive loss of weight, skin rashes, etc. At this stage the sufferer can sometimes be more ill than the 'Full-blown AIDS' sufferer and may be in need of a great deal of care and support. These symptoms may persist for many years but never develop into AIDS.

Body fluids
Term used for a number of fluids manufactured within the body that have been found to contain HIV. Though some of these fluids have been found to contain traces of the virus, not all are believed capable of transmitting HIV. The term usually refers to sperm and blood.

Butyl nitrates
See 'Poppers'.

Candida albicans
A common yeast infection, usually called 'thrush', which may occur in the vagina, or sometimes in the mouth. Severe thrush which does not respond readily to treatment may be a sign of AIDS or other types of immune deficiency disorder.

Cyclosporin
A drug commonly used after organ transplant operations to reduce the body's immune system response of rejecting foreign tissue. Controversial experimental studies have been conducted in France using cyclosporin to treat persons with AIDS.

CMV (Cytomegalovirus)
A herpes related virus which is a common cause of mononucleosis and is known to cause temporary immune disorders. CMV is believed to be associated with Kaposi's sarcoma and may play a role as an AIDS co-factor.

Co-factor
A factor or group of factors in addition to the presence of HIV that some believe may play a role in the development of AIDS. Among such co-factors may be: repeated infections with sexually transmitted diseases, and use of certain recreational drugs.

Contagious
Transmission of a disease by direct intimate contact with an infected person.

Cryptococcus neoformans

A fungus that causes a rare form of meningitis, and is now often seen as an opportunistic infection in AIDS cases.

Elisa test

A type of blood test developed which indicates whether someone has been exposed to a particular virus. The test does not detect disease, but only the antibodies formed when there has been exposure to a virus. The test can be used to detect HIV antibodies and is used to screen blood supplies and to estimate the spread of the virus.

Epidemiology

The numerical study of the progress of a disease in a population.

False negative

A negative blood test in a person who has been infected. This means either that HIV antibodies have not yet been produced or have not been detected.

False positive

A positive blood test result in a patient who has not been infected but appears to show the presence of HIV antibodies. In fact there has not been any infection.

Full-blown AIDS (sometimes known as 'Frank AIDS')

The ultimate indication that the immune system is collapsing. By this time the body has been attacked by at least one life-threatening opportunistic infection or tumor. A great deal of comfort and palliative support will definitely be needed in this stage of the disease.

GUM clinics (Genito Urinary Medicine)

Present name for 'Special' or Venereal Disease clinics. See also 'STD clinics'.

Haemophilia

An inherited disease that affects the normal clotting of blood, thus leaving the individual at risk of severe bleeding. Therapeutic blood products can control the disease. Current HIV blood screening tests have greatly reduced the risk of contaminated blood. All of the blood products used to control bleeding are now being heat treated to make them safe from HIV contamination.

HIV (Human Immunodeficiency Virus)

See 'HTLV-III'.

HPA-23
A rare antiviral drug that has been studied in AIDS research for its ability to inhibit retroviral replication.

HTLV-III (Human T-Cell Lymphotrophic Virus, Type Three)
A term first used by American scientist Dr Robert Gallo for the virus identified to be the cause of AIDS. HTLV-III may be written as 'HTLV-III/LAV', combining the American and French terminology. Virus re-named 'HIV' (Human Immunodeficiency Virus).

Incubation period
The latest or silent stage of an infectious disease intervening between the moment of infection and the appearance of symptoms. In AIDS this incubation period can be from two months to five years or longer. This should not be confused with presence of HIV antibodies. This virus can be present in the body. A positive result can occur but the person may show no signs of opportunistic infection for some considerable time.

Infectious
Capable of being easily transmitted from person to person.

Interferon
A naturally occurring substance which biologically modifies the immune response. It has been used in AIDS treatment to modify the immune response and, specifically, in the treatment of the AIDS related skin cancer, Kaposi's sarcoma.

IV Drug Taking (Intravenous Drug Taking)
One of four main behavioural patterns identified as being at high risk for contracting HIV. Drug use can entail using and often sharing unsterilised needles and syringes that serve to transmit HIV. See also 'Shooting galleries'.

KS (Kaposi's Sarcoma)
A normally rare form of skin cancer, now commonly identified as an opportunistic disease affecting persons with AIDS. KS is the formal definition of AIDS used by the Centres for Disease Control (USA).

LAV (Lymphadenopathy Associated Virus)
A term first used by French scientist Dr Luc Montagnier for the virus identified to be the cause of AIDS. LAV may

be written as 'HTLV-III/LAV', combining the American and French terminology. For HIV see 'HTLV-III'.

Leucocytes
Commonly known as white blood cells, they play a major role in fighting infectious disease. Lymphocytes are one sub-class of leucocytes. The two types of white blood cells commonly associated with AIDS are the 'B' and 'T' lymphocytes.

Lymphadenopathy
A common sign of HIV infection, identified by persistent swelling of the lymph nodes.

MMWR (Morbidity and Mortality Weekly Report)
A weekly publication in the USA by the Centres for Disease Control that serves as a reference source for information on current trends in the nation's health. It is often cited for its statistics on the number of AIDS related deaths and illnesses in the USA.

Opportunistic infections
Infections caused by a variety of viruses, bacteria, fungi and protozoa that are either nor ordinarily harmful or are easily controlled by a healthy immune system. The two most common opportunistic infections seen in AIDS are Kaposi's sarcoma (see KS) and Pneumocystis carinii pneumonia (see PCP).

PCP (Pneumocystis Carinii Pneumonia)
One of two opportunistic diseases first identified by the Centres for Disease Control in the formal definition of AIDS. It is caused by a protozoan parasite and is the most common cause of death for persons with the syndrome.

PGL (Persistant Generalised Lymphadenopathy)
Condition in which there is a generalised swelling of the lymph nodes or glands caused by viral activity.

PML (Progressive Multifocal Leukoencephalopathy)
A viral infection of the brain causing gradual memory loss, and decreased concentration, co-ordination and strength. The individual can eventually lapse into a coma. PML is often seen in AIDS cases.

Poppers
Slang term for the inhalant drug amyl or butyl nitrate that is used as a sexual stimulant. Certain AIDS research

findings indicate that it may act as an immune suppressant and that chronic use may increase suscepti-bility to AIDS.

Promiscuity

'Characterised by casual association with many sexual partners' – Universal Dictionary.

PWA (Persons With AIDS)

Preferred term used for an individual who has contracted AIDS. The term is used rather than the words 'victim' or 'sufferer'.

Retrovirus

A type of virus unknown in humans until recently. The AIDS virus is a retrovirus and as such is believed to reproduce at a rapid rate.

Seronegative

A blood screening test result indicating no presence of HIV antibodies in the bloodstream.

Seropositive

A blood screening test indicating presence of HIV anti-bodies in the bloodstream. This only indicates that a person has been exposed to the virus. It is not a test for AIDS. A seropositive person does not necessarily have AIDS and is not necessarily an AIDS patient.

Shooting galleries

Slang terms for illicit operations often set up in an aban-doned building where illegal drugs, such as heroin, cocaine and amphetamines, are purchased and injected intravenously. Often as many as 50 people will receive injections with the same unsterilised needle and syringe, thus creating the potential for mass infection among IV drug users and their sexual partners.

Spermicide

A substance commonly used as a form of contraceptive because of its ability to destroy sperm cells. Laboratory experiments have indicated that spermicides may destroy the AIDS virus.

STD (Sexually Transmitted Disease) clinics

Another term for 'Special' or Venereal Disease clinics. See also 'GUM clinics'.

Suramin

A rare antibiotic drug that is being studied in AIDS research because it is believed to inhibit retroviral replication.

T cell

A type of white blood cell that is essential in the body's fight against infection.

T cell ratio

A ratio of two types of white blood cells commonly called 'helper' and 'suppressor' cells. In AIDS there is an imbalance between the number of helper and suppressor cells. In a healthy individual this ratio is about two helpers to one suppressor; in many AIDS cases this ratio is reversed because of a deficiency in the number of helper cells.

Thrush

See 'Candida albicans'.

Victim

An unhelpful term that removes all control and responsibility from people with HIV/ARC/AIDS. It increases the pain by encouraging negative images in both the carer and the person with the virus or antibodies. To be avoided.

Resources and Services

The range of AIDS services and resources in the United States and Canada at this time would more than fill a volume. It is my intent simply to identify some of the key resources that may offer significant help to pastors or to people with AIDS, their families, friends, and caregivers.

William A. Doubleday

Key Publications for Finding AIDS-Related
Resources, Services, and Information

The following resources are especially helpful for people seeking further information about AIDS-related services or resources.

Learning AIDS: An Information Resources Directory: A Publication of the American Foundation for AIDS Research (AmFAR). Distributed by R. R. Bowker, 245 W. 17th St., New York, NY 10011. $24.95. An extensive listing of educational materials and resources, including pamphlets, posters, and audio-visuals, with critical comments by an expert review panel.

GAYELLOW PAGES, The National Edition. Published annually by Renaissance House, Box 292, Village Station, New York, NY 10014.
This is an inexpensive, remarkably exhaustive list of organizations, businesses, and services for the gay and lesbian communities in the United States and Canada. The listings by state or province, and then by city, include many under "AIDS Support and Education Services." If you have difficulty locating this publication, call the publisher: (212)674–0120. 1989 edition: $8.95 (U.S.) and $10 (Canada).

121

How to Find Information About AIDS, Virginia A. Lingle and M. Sandra Wood. New York: Harrington Park Press, 1988. A well-indexed 130 pages of resources, hotlines, health department contacts, audio-visual listings, and much more.

National Religious AIDS Coalitions

The AIDS National Interfaith Network (ANIN)
ANIN is a growing and increasingly effective national interfaith organization committed to involving the religious sector in pastoral care, advocacy, education, and networking in the AIDS crisis. This coalition of religious organizations and individuals provides vital connections among laypersons and clergy involved in AIDS ministry at the local, regional, and national levels. ANIN has established an AIDS public policy advocate in Washington, D.C., who coordinates interfaith support for enlightened AIDS legislation. It has created the interfaith Families and Friends AIDS Network and maintains a computerized national interfaith referral listing of more than 10,000 pastoral caregivers. ANIN has a priority commitment to addressing AIDS/HIV issues in communities of color, working closely with religious leaders and AIDS activists in those communities. For information or membership: ANIN, c/o United Church Board for Homeland Ministries, 475 Riverside Dr., 10th floor, New York, NY 10115. (212) 870–2100.

AIDS Task Force of National Council of Churches (NCC)
This working group of the National Council of Churches has generated policy statements and a useful packet of educational materials. For further information: AIDS Task Force, Division of Church and Society, National Council of Churches of Christ, Room 572, 475 Riverside Dr., New York, NY 10115. (212)870–2421.

Denominational AIDS Contacts

Several denominations have evolved networks or designated contact persons for purposes of coordination of effort and resources in AIDS ministry. These organizations are committed to promoting AIDS service provision, education and networking at local, regional, and national levels. Most publish newsletters, sponsor periodic conferences, and generate educational materials. Most maintain human resource listings, useful for local or regional networking. Initiating communication with your denominational contact may ultimately be mutually rewarding. While undoubtedly incomplete, this list represents key contacts as of July 1989.

American Baptist Churches in the U.S.A.
Betty Miller, Chairperson of Coordinating Committee on AIDS, American Baptist Churches in the U.S.A., P.O. Box 851, Valley Forge, PA 19482–0851. (215)768–2000.

Church of the Brethren
AIDS Ministries Task Group
The Rev. Ralph G. McFadden, Brethren Health and Welfare Association, 1451 Dundee Ave., Elgin, IL 60120. (312) 742-5100.

Episcopal Church, National Headquarters
The Rev. Randolph Frew, AIDS Consultant, 815 Second Ave., New York, NY 10017. (212)867–8400.

Episcopal Church
National Episcopal AIDS Coalition
The Rev. Thaddeus Bennett, NEAC, 1511 K St., N.W., Suite 715, Washington, D.C. 20005.

Evangelical Lutheran Church in America
The Rev. Adele Resmer, 8765 West Higgins Rd., Chicago, IL 60631. (312)380–2682.

National Catholic AIDS Network
Jay Pinkerton, O.F.M., Marie Puleo, O.S.F., Co-directors, Lazzaro Center, P.O. Box 30926, New York, NY 10011–0109. (212)779–0450.

Presbyterian AIDS Network
The Rev. Jim Hedges, John Calvin Presbyterian Church, 6501 Nebraska Ave., Tampa, FL 33604. (813)236–0941.

Union of American Hebrew Congregations
Rabbi Richard Sternberger, UAHC, 2027 Massachusetts Ave.,
N.W., Washington, D.C. 20038. (202)232–4242.

United Church of Christ AIDS Network
The Rev. Bill Johnson, United Church Board for Homeland
Ministries, AIDS Program, 475 Riverside Dr., 10th floor, New
York, NY 10115. (212)870–2100.

United Methodist Church
Cathie Lyons, Health and Welfare Ministries, General Board of
Global Ministries, United Methodist Church, Room 350, 475
Riverside Dr., New York, NY 10115. (212)870–3871.

Unitarian Universalist Association
The Rev. Scott Alexander, Unitarian Universalist Association, 25
Beacon St., Boston, MA 02108–2800. (617)742–2100.

Universal Fellowship of Metropolitan Community Churches
The Rev. A. Stephen Pieters, Universal Fellowship of Metro-
politan Community Churches, 5300 Santa Monica Blvd., Los
Angeles, CA 90029. (213)464–5100.

Selected Local AIDS Religious Groups

AIDS ministries and pastoral care networks have developed in
many communities around the nation. The following list represents some of those known to be willing to share their expertise
or materials.

CHICAGO, ILLINOIS
AIDS Pastoral Care Network, 2035 North Lincoln Ave., Chicago, IL 60614. (312)975–5180.
This well-staffed program is committed to pastoral care and
education in the Chicago area.

DALLAS/FORT WORTH, TEXAS
AIDS Interfaith Network, 6525 Inwood Rd., Dallas, TX 75209.
(214)358–4724; (817)870–1937.
This network was in the forefront of AIDS-response in Dallas.

HARTFORD, CONNECTICUT
AIDS Ministries, 1335 Asylum Avenue, Hartford, CT 06105.
(203)233–4481.
A clearinghouse for materials and resources in Connecticut,
New England, and beyond.

NEW YORK, NEW YORK
AIDS Ministries Program and Interfaith Pastoral Care Service,
AIDS Resource Center, Inc., (ARC), 24 W. 30th St., New York,
NY 10001. (212)481–1270.
AIDS Resource Center is a major provider of housing for home-
less people with AIDS. It has a pastoral staff and helps to
network pastoral care on an interfaith basis throughout the New
York City area.

AIDS Chaplaincy Program, St. Luke's–Roosevelt Hospital Center, Amsterdam and 114th St., New York, NY 10025.
(212)523–2016.
One of the first AIDS chaplaincy programs in America, it is now
much involved in pastoral care training.

MOMENTUM AIDS Outreach Program, 619 Lexington Ave.,
New York, NY 10022. (212)935–2200.
Begun under the auspices of St. Peter's Lutheran Church in New
York City, this ecumenical/interfaith program provides meals,
social services, recreation, and pastoral care to a diverse spectrum of people with AIDS. Most of the feeding program is
carried out in churches and synagogues.

PASADENA, CALIFORNIA
All Saints AIDS Service Center, 132 North Euclid, Pasadena, CA
91101. (818)796–5633.
This is a major AIDS service provider with a strong pastoral
component and a parish base. Publishes a monthly journal,
Asklepios. Subscription: $17.50 per year.

SAN FRANCISCO, CALIFORNIA
AIDS Interfaith Network, 2269 Market St., #178, San Fran-
cisco, CA 94114. (415)928–HOPE.
This was one of the first interfaith networks to respond to the
AIDS crisis.

Episcopal Chaplaincy, San Francisco General Hospital, 1001 Portrero Avenue, San Francisco, CA 94110.
One of the first chaplaincy programs in the nation to respond forcefully to the AIDS crisis.

WASHINGTON, D.C.
Episcopal Caring Response to AIDS, 2025 Eye St., N.W., Suite 917, Washington, D.C. 20005. (202) 293–5290.
A highly effective organization responding to diverse aspects of the AIDS crisis in the Washington, D.C., area, and providing services to all groups, not just to those affiliated with the Episcopal church.

Selected Contacts for National Gay and Lesbian Religious Groups

Gay and lesbian denominational caucus groups continue to be an important resource in determining where compassionate and supportive pastoral care may be available in the AIDS crisis. In many communities, groups such as Dignity and Integrity and congregations of the Metropolitan Community Church have been very active in the actual delivery of pastoral care. The national contacts that follow were known as of June 1989.

Affirmation: United Methodists for Lesbian and Gay Concerns, Box 1021, Evanston, IL 60204. (312) 475–0499.

Affirmation: Gay and Lesbian Mormons, Box 26302, San Francisco, CA 94104. (415) 641–4554.

American Baptists Concerned, 870 Erie St., Oakland, CA 94610–2268. (415) 465–8652.

Axios: Eastern and Orthodox Christians, 328 W. 17th St., #4F, New York, NY 10011. (212)989–6211.

Dignity (Gay and Lesbian Catholics), Inc., 1500 Massachusetts Ave., N.W., #11, Washington, D.C. 20005. (202) 861–0017.

Emergence International: Christian Scientists Supporting Lesbians and Gay Men, Box 581, Kentfield, CA 94914–0581. (415) 485–1881.

Evangelicals Concerned, P.O. Box 5223, Evanston, IL 60204–5223. (312) 896–3018.

Friends for Lesbian and Gay Concerns, Box 222, Sumneytown, PA 18084. (215) 234–8424.

GLAD (Gay, Lesbian, and Affirming Disciples), Box 2942, South Bend, IN 46680.

Integrity (Gay and Lesbian Episcopalians and Their Friends), Inc., Box 19561, Washington, D.C. 20036–0561. (718) 720–3054.

Lutherans Concerned/North America, Box 10461, Chicago, IL 60610–0461.

National Gay Pentecostal Alliance, Box 1391, Schenechtady, NY 12301–1391. (518) 372–6001.

Presbyterians for Lesbian/Gay Concerns, c/o James Anderson, Box 38, New Brunswick, NJ 08903–0038. (201) 846–1510.

Reformed Church in America Gay Caucus, Box 8174, Philadelphia, PA 19101–8174.

Seventh Day Adventist Kinship International, Box 3840, Los Angeles, CA 90078–3840. (213) 876–2076.

Unitarian Universalist Office of Lesbian/Gay Concerns, 25 Beacon St., Boston, MA 02108. (617)742–2100.

United Church Coalition for Lesbian/Gay Concerns, 18 N. College St., Athens, OH 45701. (614)593–7301.

Universal Fellowship of Metropolitan Community Churches, 5300 Santa Monica Blvd., #304, Los Angeles, CA 90029. (213)464–5100.

World Congress of Gay and Lesbian Jewish Organizations, Box 18961, Washington, D.C. 20036.

AIDS Organizations and Hotlines

This list includes a wide range of groups and services, some with a national focus, and others with a more local constituency.

ADAPT (Association for Drug Abuse Prevention and Treatment), 85 Bergen St., Brooklyn, NY 11201. (718)834–9585.
A leading organization in the response to the drug-related aspects of AIDS.

AID Atlanta (AIDA), 811 Cypress St., Atlanta, GA 30308. (404)872–0600.
AID Atlanta has been a leader for the South and is a source of useful educational materials.

AIDS Action Committee, 661 Boylston St., Boston, MA 02116. (617)437–6200.
This organization has been in the forefront of AIDS work in New England.

AIDS Action Council, Federation of AIDS-Related Organizations (FARO), 729 8th St., S.E., Room 200, Washington, D.C. 20003. (202)547–3101.
An important lobbying and public policy organization.

AIDS Project/Los Angeles, 7362 Santa Monica Blvd., Los Angeles, CA 90046. (213)876–8951.
A leader in AIDS response to diverse demographic groups.

American Red Cross, AIDS Education Office, 1730 D Street, N.W., Washington, D.C. 20006. (202)737–8300.
An important source of educational materials, with a particular focus on the blood supply.

Black Coalition on AIDS, Box 11908, San Francisco, CA 94103. (415)822–7228.
A group concerned with the impact of AIDS on people of color.

Canadian AIDS Hotline. 800–267–7712; 800–668–AIDS; 800–267–SIDA.
The national hotline for Canada. A good source for local Canadian resources.

Centers for Disease Control, AIDS Information Office, Atlanta, GA 30333. (404)329–2891.
The U.S. government information center on AIDS and other diseases.

128

Concern for the Dying (and Living Wills), 250 West 57th St., Room 831, New York, NY 10107. (212)246–6962.
Write here for information about the Living Will and related concerns.

Gay Men's Health Crisis, 132 W. 24th St., Box 274, New York, NY 10011. Hotline: (212)807–6655.
The leader in AIDS response in New York. A source of splendid educational materials and programs.

Haitian Coalition on AIDS, 50 Court St., Room 605, Brooklyn, NY 11201. (718)855–0972.
A group concerned with the special impact of AIDS on people of Haitian origin.

Health Education Resource Organization, Inc. (HERO), 101 W. Read St., #812, Baltimore, MD 21201. (301)685–1180.
A superb local organization that has developed excellent educational materials, including many focused on drug users, poor people, or minority communities.

Hispanic AIDS Forum, % APRED, 853 Broadway, Suite 2007, New York, NY 10003. (212)870–1902.
This organization is concerned with the growing number of AIDS cases in Hispanic communities.

Hyacinth Foundation AIDS Project, 211 Livingstone Ave., New Brunswick, NJ 08901. (201)246-0204. Hotline: 800–433–0254.
A leader in AIDS response in New Jersey, where cities like Newark and Jersey City have seen huge numbers of cases among the urban poor.

Indian AIDS Hotline. 800–283–2437.
A hotline for Native Americans.

Lambda Legal Defense and Education Fund, 666 Broadway, New York, NY 10012. (212)995–8585.
A group dedicated to legal protection for gay and lesbian persons and for people with AIDS.

The NAMES Project Quilt, Box 14573, San Francisco, CA 94114. (415)863–5511.
The national headquarters of the AIDS memorial quilt which has been traveling around the country.

National AIDS Information Clearinghouse, P.O. Box 6003, Rockville, MD 20850. 800–342–AIDS.
A national informational hotline.

The National AIDS Network, 2033 M St., N.W., Suite 800, Washington, D.C. 20036. (202) 293–2437.
A network of diverse AIDS-related organizations.

National Gay and Lesbian Task Force Crisisline. 800–SOS–GAYS.
Consistently one of the most helpful hotlines.

National Hemophilia Association, 110 Greene St., Room 406, New York, NY 10012. (212)563–0211. Hotline: (212)682–5510. An organization dedicated to the needs of hemophiliacs and their loved ones and caregivers, including those who are affected by AIDS.

National Minority AIDS Council, Box 28574, Washington, D.C. 20038. (202) 544–1076.
An organization concerned about the impact of AIDS on racial and ethnic minorities.

National Native American AIDS Prevention Center, 6239 College Ave., Suite 20a, Oakland, CA 94618. (415)658–2051.
A center devoted to AIDS prevention among Native Americans.

Pediatric AIDS Hotline, Albert Einstein College of Medicine, Bronx, NY. (212)430–3333.
A leading source of information in dealing with the growing number of pediatric AIDS cases.

San Francisco AIDS Foundation, 333 Valencia St., 4th floor, San Francisco, CA 94103. (415)864–4376. Hotline: 800–FOR–AIDS.
A long-respected leader in AIDS education in San Francisco and a source for educational materials of all kinds.

Shanti Project of San Francisco, 525 Howard St., San Francisco, CA 94105. (415)777–CARE.
This organization developed early models of caregiving for people with AIDS.

Women's AIDS Network, 333 Valencia St., San Francisco, CA 94103. Hotline: (415)864–4376.

A network concerned with the growing number of women with AIDS.

State and Local Health Departments

Virtually every state and many local communities have developed governmental responses to AIDS, usually associated with the Health Department. Often they can provide information, speakers, educational materials, and referrals. Do not hesitate to call your local, regional, state, or county Health Department and ask if they have an AIDS Hotline or AIDS information officer.

Treatment Information

For people with AIDS, people who are HIV antibody positive, and their physicians, receiving information about the best and most current treatment possibilities is a very great need. Sound pastoral care in a clinical situation includes a concern for the well-informed patient and physician. The well-informed patient is better able to make wise choices about treatment options. The well-informed physician is better able to offer positive treatment possibilities. Physicians and people with AIDS have recommended the following sources of treatment information.

American Foundation for AIDS Research, *AIDS/HIV Experimental Treatment Directory*.
Annual subscription: $30 (4 issues); single copies: $10. Send check/money order to: AmFAR, 1515 Broadway, New York, NY 10036–8901. For credit card orders only, call: (212)719–0695. Only for people with AIDS/HIV with low incomes, order a free copy by calling: 800–458–5231.

BETA (Bulletin of Experimental Treatments for AIDS).
A monthly report on treatment options in laypersons' language. San Francisco AIDS Foundation, P.O. Box 6182, San Francisco, CA 94101. (415)863–AIDS. Subscription: free.

Directory of Antiviral and Immunomodulatory Therapies for AIDS (DAITA).
Highly technical. Published by CDC AIDS Weekly, P.O. Box 830409, Birmingham, AL 35283–0409. (205)991–6920; 800–633–4931. Price: $26.

PI Perspective.
Triannual report on treatment strategies. Published by Project Inform, 347 Dolores St., Suite 301, San Francisco, CA 94110. (415)558–9051; 800–334–7422 (within California), 800–822–7422 (nationwide). Subscription: free.

PWA Coalition Newsline.
A grassroots monthly newsletter. People with AIDS Coalition, 31 W. 26th St., Fifth Floor, New York, NY 10010. (212)532–0290. Subscription: free.

PWA Voice.
Quarterly newsletter by and for people with AIDS or ARC. People with AIDS, San Francisco, 519 Castro St. Box M46, San Francisco, CA 94114. Subscription: $15 (four issues); free to low income people with AIDS or ARC.

Treatment Issues (The GMHC Newsletter of Experimental AIDS Therapies).
Gay Men's Health Crisis, Department of Medical Information, 132 W. 24th St., Box 274, New York, NY 10011. Subscription: free.

Selected Bibliography

The literature about the AIDS crisis is vast and growing constantly. This bibliography attempts to offer pastors, people with AIDS and their loved ones, and the more general reader a selective and briefly annotated view of the especially relevant literature available in the United States.

Our pastoral care and our work as AIDS educators will inevitably be strengthened if we are well informed about AIDS and well able to articulate the theology that undergirds our caring and outreach. I have placed what I consider the most useful resources first. I have tried to be more inclusive with respect to explicitly religious and pastoral materials, though some books, articles, and denominational resources have undoubtedly escaped my attention. No attempt was made to include essentially clinical/medical publications.

If you are aware of additional books, articles, or resources that should be included in this listing, I would be grateful to hear of them via the publisher, Pilgrim Press.

William A. Doubleday

AIDS—Religious and Pastoral Resources:
Excellent Resources

AMOS, WILLIAM E., JR. *When AIDS Comes to Church*. Philadelphia: Westminster Press, 1988.
A solid though sometimes cautious introduction to AIDS ministry by a Baptist pastor from Florida. Includes a useful chapter on the minister's theological preparation, drawing a contrast between judgmental theology and response on the one hand and compassionate/incarnational theology and response on the other.

DOUBLEDAY, WILLIAM A. "Spiritual and Religious Issues of AIDS," and "Death, Dying, and AIDS." In Victor Gong and Norman Rudnick, eds., *AIDS: Facts and Issues*, chaps. 22 and 23. New Brunswick, N.J.: Rutgers University Press, 1986.
Two succinct and useful pastoral chapters in a broad collection of essays about the AIDS crisis.

FORTUNATO, JOHN E. *AIDS: The Spiritual Dilemma*. San Francisco: Harper & Row, 1987.
A fine personal and theological reflection about AIDS from the perspective of an articulate gay Christian.

SHELP, EARL E., and RONALD H. SUNDERLAND. *AIDS and the Church*. Philadelphia: Westminster Press, 1987.
An introduction to AIDS ministry issues, including an excellent exploration of the relationship between sin and sickness.

SNOW, JOHN. *Mortal Fear*. Cambridge: Cowley, 1987.
A wise reflection on issues of sickness and mortality in modern culture, with particular consideration of the AIDS crisis.

AIDS—General Resources: Especially Worth Owning and Sharing

AIDS: Education and Prevention 1 (Spring 1989). Guilford Publications, 72 Spring St., New York, NY 10012.
An important new quarterly journal devoted to AIDS education and prevention. Well researched and well documented with excellent bibliographic citations.

ALYSON, SASHA, ed. *You CAN Do Something About AIDS*. Boston: The Stop AIDS Project (40 Plympton St., 02118), 1988.
This widely distributed "give-away" book is full of ideas and resources about responding positively to the AIDS crisis. A wonderful source of inspiration for clergy or parishes wondering about what they can *do*.

DREUILHE, EMMANUEL. *Mortal Embrace: Living with AIDS*. New York: Hill & Wang, 1988.
A provocative reflection by a person with AIDS, openly critical of many religious leaders.

FEE, ELIZABETH, and DANIEL M. FOX, eds. *AIDS: The Burden of History*. Berkeley: University of California Press, 1988.

An impressive anthology exploring the historical and cultural significance of the AIDS epidemic.

GONG, VICTOR, and NORMAN RUDNICK, eds. *AIDS: Facts and Issues*. New Brunswick, N.J.: Rutgers University Press, 1986.
A solid collection of essays, although the medical chapters are beginning to be dated.

"Living With AIDS." *Daedalus, Journal of the American Academy of Arts and Sciences,* two-part special issue. 118, Numbers 2 and 3 (Spring and Summer 1989). $12 from *Daedalus* Business Office, P.O. Box 515, Canton, MA 02021.
A collection of excellent articles by recognized leaders in various aspects of AIDS response. Virtually every article includes a valuable and usually exhaustive bibliography.

SABATIER, RENEE. *Blaming Others: Prejudice, Race and Worldwide AIDS*. London: Panos Institute, 1988.
A provocative exploration of the AIDS crisis throughout the world, with particular attention given to issues of race and prejudice.

Scientific American 259 (October 1988). "What Science Knows About AIDS." A single-topic issue.
An excellent survey/summary of the scientific knowledge as of mid-1988. Since published as a paperback reprint.

SHILTS, RANDY. *And the Band Played On: Politics, People, and the AIDS Epidemic*. New York: St. Martin's Press, 1987.
An exhaustive chronological account of the AIDS epidemic.

AIDS—Religious and Pastoral Resources:
Extensive Listing

BECHTEL, DANIEL R. "The Bible and AIDS: An Example of Biblical Perspectives Informing Modern Theology and Ethics." *Prism: A Theological Forum for the UCC* 12 (Spring 1987): 66–78.
A helpful examination of hermeneutical issues raised by the AIDS crisis.

BISHOP, JOSEPH P. *Soul Mending: Letters to Friends in Crisis*. Wilton, Conn.: Morehouse-Barlow, 1986. 143–65.

A wise pastor writes letters to his friends in crisis, including a mother and her son facing death in the AIDS crisis.

BLAXTON, REGINALD G. "Will Church Punish or Heal?" *The Witness* 70 (October 1987): 20–22.
An Episcopal priest, a person of color, who serves on the staff of the mayor of Washington, D.C., reflects on the AIDS crisis.

CASTRO, R. MICHAEL. "AIDS and the Ministry of the Church." Pamphlet published in 1987 by United Methodist Discipleship Resources, P.O. Box 842, Nashville, TN 37202.
A pamphlet aimed at Methodist congregations and pastors.

Christianity and Crisis 48 (July 4, 1988): "A Special Issue: AIDS."
An excellent collection of current articles. A great resource for an adult education class.

Christianity Today (August 7, 1987). "Ministry in Plague Time: Will the Church Stand Behind Those Who Have AIDS?" pp. 15–22.
An attempt at a compassionate evangelical response.

FLYNN, EILEEN P. *AIDS: A Catholic Call for Compassion.* Kansas City: Sheed & Ward, 1985.
An early Roman Catholic contribution to pastoral response.

———. *Teaching About AIDS.* Kansas City: Sheed & Ward, 1988.
Aimed at teaching young people about AIDS, this book is *very limited* in usefulness due to its very traditional moral theology and its opposition to teaching about "safer" forms of sexual behavior.

GALLAGHER, JOSEPH. *Voices of Strength and Hope for a Friend with AIDS.* Kansas City: Sheed & Ward, 1987.
A Roman Catholic priest offers a collection of hopeful spiritual resources for people with AIDS.

HALLMAN, DAVID G., ed. *AIDS Issues: Confronting the Challenge.* New York: Pilgrim Press, 1989.
A collection of short conference papers on various aspects of the AIDS crisis.

HANCOCK, LEE. "Fear and Healing in the AIDS Crisis." *Christianity and Crisis* (June 24, 1985): 255–58.
An important early article by one of the women in the forefront of pastoral response to AIDS.

HORRIGAN, ALICE. "AIDS and the Catholic Church." In *The Social Impact of AIDS in the U.S.,* edited by Richard A. Berk, 83–

113. Cambridge: Abt Books, 1988.
An excellent article on the Catholic church with special attention to AIDS cases in the Latino community.

JURGENSON, STANLEY D., and LYLE GREINER. "Pastoral Care to AIDS Victim." *Specialized Pastoral Care Journal* 8 (1986): 23–27.
Despite its use of "victim" language, it includes some useful common-sense pastoral care advice.

KAYAL, PHILIP M. " 'Morals,' Medicine, and the AIDS Epidemic." *Journal of Religion and Health* 24 (Fall 1985): 218–38.
A sociological exploration of the role of religion in the AIDS crisis.

Lutheran Social Services of Northern California. "AIDS Resources for Congregations."
A resource packet available for $17.45 (including postage) from LSS, 1101 O'Farrell St., San Francisco, CA 94109.
The materials include articles, curricular tools, and quick reference information.

MILLER, GLENN T. "Ministerial Ethics and AIDS." *The Christian Ministry* (May 1986): 22–24.
A brief, helpful article that raises issues of ministerial/professional ethics.

MILLIKEN, WESTON, and PAUL STEARNS. *Proceedings of the Interfaith Conference on AIDS and ARC, San Francisco, March 21–22, 1987.* San Francisco: Interfaith Conference Steering Committee, 1988.
Proceedings of a conference that reflected a broad ecumenical and interfaith dimension in the San Francisco area.

Mission Discoveries. Report #9, March 1986: "AIDS: A Challenge to the Church." Division for Service and Mission in America, American Lutheran Church.
A fine effort to raise AIDS issues in the Lutheran church.

Mission Discoveries. Report #12, July 1987: "AIDS: A Serious and Special Opportunity for Ministry." Division for Service and Mission in America, American Lutheran Church.
A follow-up to the above publication.

Moody Monthly 89 (October 1988): "AIDS—Can We Only Condemn?" pp. 16–29.
Several articles representing a conservative Christian response.

MURPHY, PATRICE. "Pastoral Care and Persons with AIDS." *American Journal of Hospice Care* (March/April 1986): 38–40.
The views of a compassionate Roman Catholic religious who has been involved in AIDS pastoral care almost from the beginning.

National Catholic Reporter.
. Offers regular coverage of the AIDS crisis from a liberal Catholic perspective.

NELSON, JAMES B. "Responding to, Learning from AIDS." *Christianity and Crisis* (May 19, 1986): 176–81.
An important and comprehensive article by a leading liberal Protestant theologian of human sexuality.

Open Hands: Journal of the Reconciling Congregation Program. (Summer 1988): special issue: "AIDS and the Church." $5.75 per issue from P.O. Box 23636, Washington, D.C. 20026.
This quarterly journal addresses gay and lesbian concerns in the Methodist and other Protestant churches.

PHILLIPS, JENNIFER M. "The Future of AIDS: Parishes Can Help." *Christian Century* (June 1, 1988): 548–51.
A succinct view of ways parishes can get involved.

Religious Education 83 (Spring 1988): "AIDS: Sexual Responsibility and Ethics." 409 Prospect St., New Haven, CT 06511–2177.
A rich collection of varied articles exploring sexual ethics, AIDS education, and related issues.

SCHAPER, RICHARD L. "Pastoral Care for Persons with AIDS and for Their Families." *Christian Century* (August 12–19, 1987): 691–94.
A succinct and useful article in a journal that has offered steady and helpful AIDS coverage.

SHELP, EARL E., and RONALD H. SUNDERLAND. "AIDS and the Church." *Christian Century* (September 11–18, 1985).
A landmark early article followed by their several books.

———. *AIDS: A Manual for Pastoral Care.* Philadelphia: Westminster Press, 1987.
A practical guide to basic pastoral care issues for beginning pastors.

SHELP, EARL E., RONALD H. SUNDERLAND, and PETER W. A. MANSELL. *AIDS: Personal Stories in Pastoral Perspective.* New York:

Pilgrim Press, 1986.
Through personal stories—mostly of gay men—readers are offered a way to begin to comprehend the pain and complexity of the AIDS crisis.

SIDER, RONALD J. "AIDS: An Evangelical Perspective." *Christian Century* (January 6–13, 1988): 11–14.
A sincere attempt to state a simultaneously compassionate and essentially conservative Evangelical position regarding AIDS.

SMITH, WALTER J. *AIDS: Living and Dying with Hope: Issues in Pastoral Care.* New York: Paulist Press, 1988.
A thoughtful book by a compassionate Roman Catholic.

STILES, B. J. "AIDS and the Churches." *Christianity and Crisis* (January 13, 1986): 534–36.
An important call to further action by a theologically trained AIDS activist.

TILLERAAS, PERRY. *The Color of Light: Meditations for All of Us Living with AIDS.* San Francisco: Harper & Row, 1988.
Inspired by the Hazelden Foundation, this book offers an inspirational passage for each day.

WINDAL, CLAUDIA. "The Way of the Cross for Persons with AIDS." *Witness* 69 (September 1986): 16–17.
An adaptation of the Stations of the Cross to the AIDS crisis.

Aids—Religious and Pastoral Response: Dangerous

ADAMS, MOODY. *AIDS: You Just Think You're Safe.* Baker, La.: Dalton Moody, 1986.
A frightening example of extremely conservative Christian hatemongering and misinformation.

ANTONIO, GENE. *The AIDS Cover-Up? The Real and Alarming Facts About AIDS.* San Francisco: Ignatius Press, 1986.
Another version of judgmental theology combined with fearful medical misinformation.

CHILTON, DAVID. *Power in the Blood: A Christian Response to AIDS.* Brentwood, Tenn.: Wolgemuth & Hyatt, 1987.
A strongly homophobic view of the AIDS crisis combined with a misguided interest in healing ministries.

AIDS: Ethical and Legal Issues

AIDS and the Law: A Guide for the Public. Edited by Harlon L. Dalton, Scott Burris, and the Yale AIDS Law Project. New Haven: Yale University Press, 1987.
A broad exploration of legal issues raised by the AIDS crisis.

Bulletin of the Park Ridge Center. 676 N. St. Clair, Suite 450, Chicago, IL 60611.
The bulletin is published about three times a year and has included considerable discussion and bibliography about AIDS.

Hastings Center Report (December 1986): special supplement: "AIDS: Public Health and Civil Liberties." 36 pages. $6.00.

Hastings Center Report (April/May 1988): special supplement: "AIDS: The Responsibilities of Health Professionals." 32 pages. $4.00. Available from Publications Department, The Hastings Center, 255 Elm Road, Briarcliff Manor, NY 10510.
The Hastings Center is the leading medical ethics research group in America. Its *Report* regularly covers AIDS issues.

MURPHY, TIMOTHY F. "Is AIDS a Just Punishment?" *Journal of Medical Ethics* (London) 14 (1988):154–60.
Murphy, a professor of biomedical sciences at the University of Illinois, considers the notion of AIDS as a punishment.

PIERCE, CHRISTINE, and DONALD VANDEVEER, eds. *AIDS: Ethics and Public Policy.* Belmont, Calif.: Wadsworth Publishing Co., 1988.
A solid collection of essays to support ethical discussion or education.

Second Opinion. Published by the Park Ridge Center, 676 N. St. Clair, Suite 450, Chicago, IL 60611.
A quarterly publication which explores issues of faith, health, suffering, ethics, and related concerns. Many articles in recent years have had implications for care in the AIDS crisis.

AIDS: General Resources

ALTMAN, DENNIS. *AIDS in the Mind of America.* New York: Doubleday & Co., 1987.
A cultural analysis of the AIDS crisis by a distinguished gay sociologist.

BERK, RICHARD A., ed. *The Social Impact of AIDS in the U.S.* Cambridge: Abt Books, 1988.
An excellent cross section of articles on various psychological and sociological aspects of the AIDS crisis.

CRIMP, DOUGLAS, ed. *AIDS: Cultural Analysis/Cultural Activism.* Cambridge: MIT Press, 1988.
An uneven collection of essays exploring the sociocultural implications and possibilities of the AIDS crisis.

FELDMAN, DOUGLAS A., and THOMAS M. JOHNSON, eds. *The Social Dimensions of AIDS.* New York: Frederick A. Praeger, 1986.
A rich anthology exploring the diverse social dimensions of the AIDS crisis.

KUBLER-ROSS, ELISABETH. *AIDS: The Ultimate Challenge.* New York: Macmillan Co., 1987.
A surprisingly disappointing book by one of the true pioneers in work with the dying; it seems pasted together and poorly structured.

LANGONE, JOHN. *AIDS: The Facts.* Boston: Little, Brown, & Co., 1988.
A readable nonsensationalized journalistic overview of the epidemic.

MONETTE, PAUL. *Borrowed Time: An AIDS Memoir.* San Diego: Harcourt Brace Jovanovich, 1988.
A moving account of a friend's illness by a distinguished gay novelist.

NORWOOD, CHRIS. *Advice for Life: A Woman's Guide to AIDS Risks and Prevention.* New York: Pantheon Books, 1987.
One of several AIDS books with an emphasis on women's concerns.

PEABODY, BARBARA. *The Screaming Room: A Mother's Journal of Her Son's Struggle with AIDS.* San Diego: Oak Tree Publications, 1986.
A moving account of a mother's love and struggle.

RICHARDSON, DIANE. *Women and AIDS.* New York: Methuen, Inc., 1988.
An excellent resource for those working with women at risk for AIDS.

SCHINAZI, RAYMOND F., and ANDRE J. NAHMIAS, eds. *AIDS in Children, Adolescents and Heterosexual Adults: An Interdisciplinary*

Approach to Prevention. New York: Elsevier, 1988.
This large volume is the outgrowth of a conference in 1987 and is not very readable.

Social Casework: The Journal of Contemporary Social Work 69 (June 1988): special issue: "AIDS: Bridging the Gap between Information and Practice."
A contemporary social-work-oriented collection of articles.

SONTAG, SUSAN. *AIDS and Its Metaphors.* New York: Farrar, Straus & Giroux, 1989.
The author of *Illness as Metaphor* offers her own much talked about but unextraordinary view of the AIDS crisis.

TURNER, CHARLES, HEATHER MILLER, AND LINCOLN MOSES, eds. *AIDS, Sexual Behavior, and Intravenous Drug Use.* Washington, D.C.: National Academy Press, 1989.
An important compilation of materials regarding AIDS and the drug user.

WHITMORE, GEORGE. *Someone Was Here: Profiles in the AIDS Epidemic.* New York: New American Library, 1988.
Offers profiles of people living with and/or dying with AIDS.

Healing

There is a growing literature of psychological and spiritual healing that some people with AIDS and their pastors have found helpful. Those interested in finding healing resources for the AIDS crisis may find the following resources helpful.

BAKKEN, KENNETH L., and KATHLEEN H. HOFELLER. *The Journey Toward Wholeness: A Christ-Centered Approach to Health and Healing.* New York: Crossroad, 1988.

COUSINS, NORMAN. *The Healing Heart.* New York: Avon Books, 1983.

FINK, PETER E., ed. *Alternative Futures for Worship.* Vol. 7, *Anointing of the Sick.* Collegeville, Minn.: Liturgical Press, 1987.

HAY, LOUISE. *You Can Heal Your Life.* Santa Monica: Hay House, 1984.

KELSEY, MORTON T. *Psychology, Medicine, and Christian Healing.* San Francisco: Harper & Row, 1988.

LINN, DENNIS, and MATTHEW LINN. *Healing of Memories.* New York: Paulist Press, 1974.

MADDOCKS, MORRIS. *The Christian Healing Ministry*. London: SPCK, 1981.

MARTY, MARTIN. "Religion and Healing: The Four Expectations." *Second Opinion* 7 (March 1988): 61–80.

SEYBOLD, KLAUS, and ULRICH B. MUELLER. *Sickness and Healing*. Biblical Encounters Series. Nashville: Abingdon Press, 1981.

SIEGEL, BERNIE S. *Love, Medicine and Miracles*. New York: Harper & Row, 1986.

SIMONTON, CARL, and STEPHANIE SIMONTON. *Getting Well Again*. New York: J. B. Tarcher, 1978.

Death, Dying, Grief, and Bereavement

GENTLES, IAN, ed. *Care for the Dying and the Bereaved*. Toronto: Anglican Book Center, 1982.

GOLDBERG, JACOB. *Pastoral Bereavement Counseling: A Structured Program to Help Mourners*. New York: Human Sciences Press, 1989.

KUBLER-ROSS, ELISABETH. *On Death and Dying*. New York: Macmillan Co., 1969.

———, ed. *Death: The Final Stage of Growth*. Englewood Cliffs, N.J.: Prentice-Hall, 1975.

KUSHNER, HAROLD S. *When Bad Things Happen to Good People*. New York: Avon Books, 1981.

MEYER, CHARLES. *Surviving Death: A Practical Guide to Caring for the Dying and Bereaved*. Mystic, Conn.: Twenty-Third Publications, 1988.

MUNLEY, ANNE. *The Hospice Alternative*. New York: Basic Books, 1983.

PLATT, LARRY A., and ROGER G. BRANCH. *Resources for Ministry in Death and Dying*. Nashville: Broadman, 1988.

RANDO, THERESE A. *Grief, Dying, and Death*. Champaign, Ill.: Research Press, 1984.

SANDERS, CATHERINE M. *Grief: The Mourning After. Dealing With Adult Bereavement*. New York: John Wiley and Sons, 1989.

WORDEN, J. WILLIAM. *Grief Counseling and Grief Therapy*. New York: Springer Publishing, 1982.

Human Sexuality and Theology

Work with the AIDS crisis in the church often stimulates the need to go further in one's theological reflection on human sexuality. I have found these resources especially helpful in evolving a compassionate and inclusive theology and psychology of human sexuality.

BOSWELL, JOHN. *Christianity, Social Tolerance, and Homosexuality.* Chicago: University of Chicago Press, 1980.

BROWN, PETER. *The Body and Society: Men, Women, and Sexual Renunciation in Early Christianity.* New York: Columbia University Press, 1988.

BRUNDAGE, JAMES A. *Law, Sex, and Christian Society in Medieval Europe.* Chicago: University of Chicago Press, 1987.

CAHILL, LISA SOWLE. *Between the Sexes: Foundations for a Christian Ethics of Sexuality.* Philadelphia: Fortress Press, 1985.

COUNTRYMAN, L. WILLIAM. *Dirt, Greed, and Sex: Sexual Ethics in the New Testament and Their Implications for Today.* Philadelphia: Fortress Press, 1988.

D'EMILIO, JOHN, and ESTELLE B. FREEDMAN. *Intimate Matters: A History of Sexuality in America.* New York: Harper & Row, 1988.

EDWARDS, GEORGE R. *Gay/Lesbian Liberation.* New York: Pilgrim Press, 1984.

FORTUNATO, JOHN E. *Embracing the Exile: Healing Journeys of Gay Christians.* New York: Seabury Press, 1982.

FRIEDMAN, RICHARD C. *Male Homosexuality: A Contemporary Psychoanalytic Perspective.* New Haven: Yale University Press, 1988.

GOERGEN, DONALD. *The Sexual Celibate.* New York: Seabury Press, 1974.

GREENBERG, DAVID F. *The Construction of Homosexuality.* Chicago: University of Chicago Press, 1988.

HANIGAN, JAMES P. *Homosexuality: The Test Case for Christian Sexual Ethics.* New York: Paulist Press, 1988.

ISAY, RICHARD A. *Being Homosexual: Gay Men and Their Development.* New York: Farrar, Straus & Giroux, 1989.

KOSNIK, ANTHONY, et al. *Human Sexuality: New Directions in Catholic Moral Thought.* New York: Paulist Press, 1977.

MARMOR, JUDD, ed. *Homosexual Behavior*. New York: Basic Books, 1980.

McNEILL, JOHN J. *The Church and the Homosexual*. Kansas City: Sheed, Andrews, McMeel, 1976.

MINTZ, STEVEN and SUSAN KELLOGG. *Domestic Revolutions: A Social History of American Family Life*. New York: Free Press, 1988.

MOHR, RICHARD D. *Gays and Justice: A Study of Ethics, Society, and the Law*. New York: Columbia University Press, 1988.

NELSON, JAMES B. *Embodiment: An Approach to Sexuality and Christian Theology*. Minneapolis: Augsburg Publishing House, 1978.

———. *The Intimate Connection: Male Sexuality, Masculine Spirituality*. Philadelphia: Westminster Press, 1988.

PITTENGER, NORMAN. *Making Sexuality Human*. New York: Pilgrim Press, 1970.

RUSE, MICHAEL. *Homosexuality: A Philosophical Inquiry*. New York: Basil Blackwell & Mott, 1988.

SCANZONI, LETHA, and VIRGINIA R. MOLLENKOTT. *Is the Homosexual My Neighbor?* San Francisco: Harper & Row, 1978.

SCROGGS, ROBIN. *The New Testament and Homosexuality*. Philadelphia: Fortress Press, 1983.

SPONG, JOHN SHELBY. *Living in Sin: A Bishop Rethinks Human Sexuality*. San Francisco: Harper & Row, 1988.

The United Church of Christ. *Human Sexuality: A Preliminary Study*. New York: United Church Press, 1977.

WEINRICH, JAMES D. *Sexual Landscapes*. New York: Charles Scribner's Sons, 1987.